INTEGRATION AND COORDINATION OF METABOLIC PROCESSES

A Systems Approach to Endocrinology

INTEGRATION AND COORDINATION OF METABOLIC PROCESSES

A Systems Approach to Endocrinology

J. H. U. Brown, Ph. D.
Coordinator
Southwest Research Consortium

VAN NOSTRAND REINHOLD COMPANY
NEW YORK CINCINNATI ATLANTA DALLAS SAN FRANCISCO
LONDON TORONTO MELBOURNE

Van Nostrand Reinhold Company Regional Offices:
New York   Cincinnati   Atlanta   Dallas   San Francisco

Van Nostrand Reinhold Company International Offices:
London   Toronto   Melbourne

Copyright © 1978 by Litton Educational Publishing, Inc.

Library of Congress Catalog Card Number: 77-25817
ISBN: 0-442-20940-1

All rights reserved. No part of this work covered by the copyright hereon may be reproduced or used in any form or by any means—graphic, electronic, or mechanical, including photocopying, recording, taping, or information storage and retrieval systems—without permission of the publisher.

Manufactured in the United States of America

Published by Van Nostrand Reinhold Company
135 West 50th Street, New York, N.Y. 10020

Published simultaneously in Canada by Van Nostrand Reinhold Ltd.

15 14 13 12 11 10 9 8 7 6 5 4 3 2 1

Library of Congress Cataloging in Publication Data

Brown, Jack Harold Upton, 1918–
  Integration and coordination of metabolic processes.

  Includes bibliographies and index.
  1. Endocrinology.   2. Metabolic regulation.
I. Title.
QP187.B646   599'.01'927   77-25817
ISBN 0-442-20940-1

Preface

It requires some temerity for an author to attempt to write a book on endocrinology, when many volumes on the market have approached the subject carefully and well. The only excuse is one of a different approach. Endocrinology can be approached, as in so many books, from the standpoint of each individual gland and the mechanisms of health and disease that are affected by that gland. It is the author's contention that such an approach neglects the more important aspects of endocrinology, the integration of all activities of the body into a single unified whole, which we call *homeostasis*. An understanding must be obtained of the control systems, and of how the endocrine glands both operate in controlling bodily functions and are themselves controlled, either by higher nervous centers, or by feedback from the body itself. It is important to understand that control of carbohydrate, protein, and fat metabolism is a function of the endocrine glands and their interrelationships with each other, and so a knowledge of integration of endocrine activity is extremely important to an understanding of how the endocrine glands function in health and disease. This book attempts to provide some of this knowledge. The readers will find in this text information about the anatomy and physiology of the endocrine glands, because this is important to understanding overall functions. They will, moreover, find material that is not usually included in the standard endocrine text.

In this volume, control diagrams outline the way in which the endocrine glands function in relation to themselves and to each other. There are many diagrams showing the integrated response of the endocrine glands on control of carbohydrate, protein, and fat metabolism. Because this is a new approach to endocrinology, there has been little attempt to document each individual piece of information with citations from the literature. Rather, the author has attempted to provide those references that will give an overview of the situation, and permit the readers to delve further, as they see fit. An attempt has been made to include references through 1975, which in themselves contain additional references leading the reader back into the history of some particular phenomenon. In some cases, where it is believed that the historical information is important, the earlier references have been included. The works of Berson and Yalow on RIAs and of Verney on osmoreceptors have been included solely for this reason. Finally, diseases of the endocrine organs have been included and mentioned only where the metabolic consequences are important and can be related to an overall integration of function. No attempt has been made to define the individual clinical syndromes and the clinical findings that occur.

Modern approaches to endocrinology demand a knowledge of control theory and cybernetics because they are the basis of endocrine function. We have done our best to provide this information, although many glands have not been satisfactorily investigated from this viewpoint. Similarly, the coupling between many of the endocrines is not clear-cut. The information available does make a new viewpoint possible, which will, it is hoped, add to an understanding of how metabolic processes are integrated.

It is the hope of the author that the reader will find this book a guide to the integrative study of the endocrine gland. The author will welcome criticism, in case there is another edition.

Acknowledgments

The author wishes to express grateful appreciation to Dr. Dyke Kalu, Department of Physiology, University of Texas Health Science Center at San Antonio, for many hours spent in review of the manuscript and for many helpful suggestions.

Thanks are also extended to F. A. Davis Co. for permission to use material from a previous textbook, and to the publisher for forbearance in what is always a difficult task.

A List of Common Abbreviations in Endocrinology

ACTH	Adrenocorticotrophic hormone, corticotrophin
ADH	Antidiuretic hormone, vasopressin
APL	Anterior pituitarylike hormone
AZ	Ascheim-Zondek pregnancy test
BMR	Basal metabolic rate
CRF	Corticortrophin-releasing factor
EPF	Exophthalmos-producing factor
FSH	Follicle-stimulating hormone
GH	Growth hormone (also STH)
HCG	Human chorionic gonadotrophin
IF	Inhibitory factors (PIF—prolactin inhibitory factors)
ICSH	Interstitial cell-stimulating hormone (see LH)
LATS	Long-acting thyroid stimulator
LH	Luteinizing hormone; same material as ICSH
LTH	Luteotrophic hormone; luteotrophin, prolactin, lactogenic hormone
MSH	Melanocyte-stimulating hormone
NEFA	Nonesterified fatty acids (also FFA, fatty acids)
NPH	Neutral protamine Hagedorn insulin (long-acting)

PBI	Protein-bound iodine
PMS	Pregnant mare serum
PTH	Parathyroid hormone (parathormone)
PZI	Protamine zinc insulin
RIA	Radioimmunoassay
RF	Releasing factors (such as TRF, GRF, CRF, etc.)
STH	Somatotrophic (growth) hormone
T_3	Triiodothyronine (also TRIT)
T_4	Thyroxine
TBP	Thyroxine-binding protein (TBG—thyroxine-binding globulin; TBPA—thyroxine-binding prealbumin)
T/S	Thyroid-to-serum-iodine ratio, determined with I^{131}
TSH	Thyroid-stimulating hormone, thyrotrophin
USP	U.S. Pharmacopeia

Contents

Preface   v
Acknowledgments   vii
A List of Common Abbreviations in Endocrinology   ix

1. Introduction   1

　Actions of the Hormones   2
　Proof of Existence of a Hormone   4
　Other Considerations   5
　Secretion, Transport, and Excretion   8
　Hormone Assay   9
　Homeokinesis   11
　The Form of Hormones   12

2. Control Processes in Nature   14

　Amplification, or Gain, of a Control System   15
　Transfer Functions   16
　　General Analysis of a Control System   17
　　More Complex Analysis of a Control System   17
　　Steady-State Versus Transient Analysis of Control Systems   18
　Oscillation of Control Systems   19
　Rhythms in Biological Activity   20
　Remarks on Control in the Endocrine System   26
　References   27

3. The Cellular Activity of Hormones   29

Site of Action of the Hormones   30
The Role of Receptors   33
Assay of Receptors   35
Hormonal Interrelationships   36
References   41

4. The Pituitary and the Hypothalamus   42

The Pituitary   42
  Anatomy   43
  Histology   43
The Hormones of the Anterior Pituitary   45
  Activity of the Trophic Hormones   46
  Control of Growth Hormone   50
TSH   55
Adrenocorticotrophin (ACTH)   56
  Gonadotrophins   58
    FSH   59
    LH   60
    LTH   60
    Chorionic Gonadotrophin   61
The Hypothalamus   62
  Secretion of Anterior Pituitary Hormones   62
  Portal System of the Pituitary   62
  Hypothalamic Mechanism and Mediator   65
    CRF   67
    TSH   67
References   68

5. Neurohypophysis and Other Hormonal Agents   70

Hormone Production   71
  The Oxytocic Hormone   73
  Vasopressin-Antidiuretic Hormone   74
The Intermediate Lobe   78
The Pineal Lobe   80
The Prostaglandins   82
References   85

6. The Thyroid   87

Iodine Metabolism   88
The Thyroid Hormone   93
   The Circulating Thyroid Hormone   95
   Metabolism of Thyroid Hormones   97
   Control of Thyroid Secretion   98
Activity of the Thyroid Hormone   101
Antithyroid Drugs   105
The Thyroid and Other Endocrine Organs   106
Tests of Thyroid Function   107
References   109

7. The Adrenal Gland   110

The Adrenal Cortex   111
   Control of the Adrenal Cortex   112
   The Adrenal Steroids   116
   Metabolic Paths   119
Metabolic Effects of Adrenocortical Hormones   124
   Salt and Water Metabolism   126
   Other Effects of Adrenalectomy   128
   Assay of Corticoids   131
   Stress and the Adrenal Cortex   132
References   133

8. The Adrenal Medulla   134

Hormones of the Adrenal Medulla   134
   Activity of Medullary Hormones   136
   Assay of Catecholamines   140
References   141

9. Calcium Metabolism: Parathyroid Hormone and Thyrocalcitonin   142

Parathyroid Hormone   142
The Bone   143
Control of Calcium Level   144
Vitamin D   147
Calcium and Phosphorus Metabolism   150
Metabolic Effects of Parathyroids   154

Thyrocalcitonin   155
References   156

10. The Pancreas   157

Carbohydrate Metabolism   158
Insulin   160
   Insulin Activity: Effects of Insulin Lack   161
   Site of Action of Insulin   165
   Control of Insulin Secretion   167
   Innervation of the Pancreas   169
   Other Insulin Effects   170
      Interrelationships of the Pancreas   171
      Oversecretion and Undersecretion   174
Oral Hypoglycemic Agents   174
Hyperglycemic Agents   175
Diabetes Mellitus   177
Endocrine Control of Energy Sources   179
   General Metabolic Controls   181
   Exercise   183
   Mobilization of Energy Sources   183
References   184

11. Endocrinology of the Male   186

The Testes   186
   Function of the Testes   187
The Androgens   187
The Androgens as Sex Hormones   190
   Control of Hormone Secretion   191
Interrelations Between the Testes and Other Organ Systems   194
   Extrasexual Activity of Androgens   195
References   196

12. Endocrinology of the Female   197

The Ovary   197
   The Ovarian Follicle   197
The Female Sex Hormones   199
   The Estrogens and Progesterone   199
   Influence of Estrogens on Metabolic Processes   202
   Control of Ovarian Function   202

The Menstrual Cycle 206
Estrogens as Sex Hormones 210
Effects of Estrogen on Other Hormones 211
Failure of Ovarian Secretion 212
   Progesterone 212
Pregnancy 214
Parturition and Lactation 218
   Theories Regarding Initiation of Parturition 218
   Relaxin 219
   Lactation 220
References 211

Appendix 222

   Control System 222
   References 225

Index 227

1
Introduction

Endocrinology is a science that cannot properly be placed in any single one of the recognized medical subdivisions since it so widely overlaps and enters into them all. The endocrinologist must be an anatomist to understand the production of hormones in specific cell types, a biochemist to determine the structure of the material, a physiologist to ascertain the function of a gland or hormone, a pathologist to investigate the effects of the hormones, and a pharmacologist to appreciate therapeutic implications and the importance of possible side effects.

One of the major difficulties in entering upon any field is the problem of definition. In no field of endeavor is this so difficult as in endocrinology. *Endocrinology* stresses internal secretion as opposed to external, as in the case of the pancreas, and is derived from *endo* (Greek, "within") plus *krinein* (Greek, "to separate"). The word *hormone* coined in 1905 by Ernest Starling for the substance *secretin*, was taken from the Greek word meaning "to excite" because secretin caused the production of typical products from the intestinal and pancreatic mucosa. Since that time, the word *hormone* has been adapted to many uses. For example, carbon dioxide excites the cells of the respiratory center, and some workers have proposed this substance as a hormone. In the discussions herein, we will retain the classical definition as modified in the following paragraphs.

Current thinking has resulted in general acceptance of the proposal of Sir William Bayliss and Ernest Starling that a hormone be defined as "any substance normally produced by specialized cells in some part of the body and carried to other parts by the blood stream where it affects the body as a whole."

The author is using another definition: *Endocrinology is the study of those processes designed to transfer information for the control of bodily processes as an integrated system.* Under this definition, a hormone is a substance that acts as an agent of communication and control, which is a broader definition than that under the classical approach. This definition also lends itself better to applications in control theory. In many ways, it is thoroughly satisfactory as it brings into prominence the idea of *homeokinesis*,* the dynamic maintenance of the constant body environment that is so necessary for survival, because most of the hormones are catalysts—that is, they do not initiate a reaction but modify rate processes in the body even though the change in rate may be great.

The body must be able to transfer information from one part of the system to another for protection, nutrition, and a host of other processes. The information transfer is accomplished through a *fast* system (the nervous system) and a *slow* system (the endocrines). The overall physiological actions of the hormones may be lumped under the general headings of coordination, transport, material utilization, synthesis, and growth.

ACTIONS OF THE HORMONES

Before we can begin to examine the functions of the hormones, we must make a series of generalizations that apply to most hormones and without which many of the hormonal actions will not be clear. It has been suggested that the hormones are able to modify enzyme processes in the cell (thyroxine), affect the rate of transfer of material across the cell wall (insulin), or alter the physical relationships of subcellular components (thyroid-stimulating hormone, TSH). It is well known that many hormones have a great specificity; the action of TSH on the thyroid, of adrenocorticotrophin (ACTH) on the adrenal cortex, and of estrogen, testosterone, and the gonadotrophins on the sex organs are excellent examples. On the other hand,

---

*The author is making this break from the traditional *homeostasis*, coined by Walter Cannon to emphasize the nonstatic nature of the equilibrium apparent in most biological systems.

the adrenal steroids, thyroid hormones, and others appear to act on a wide variety of cells in the body.

The hormones perform three major functions in the body, and almost all endocrine functions can be grouped under one of them.

1. *Integrative action.* By traveling in the bloodstream and reaching all cells of the body, the hormones permit the body to act as a whole in response to external or internal stimuli. This is clearly seen in reactions of fright or stress.
2. *Regulation.* The action of the hormones in regulating the internal environment has been stressed time and again, and examples are numerous. The regulation of salt and water balance, metabolism, and growth may be mentioned.
3. *Morphogenesis.* Some hormones play an important part in controlling the rate and type of growth of the organism. The development of male and female sex characteristics and the rate of growth of the various parts of the body and their relative size relationships appear to be under endocrine control.

The endocrine organs may be arbitrarily divided into two major types on the basis of their products:

1. The trophic hormones produced mainly by the pituitary and hypothalamus, which stimulate and maintain certain other endocrine glands.* The target glands are unable to maintain a normal rate of secretion in the absence of the trophic hormones although the process does not completely cease.
2. Hormones secreted by glands other than the pituitary. The term *target organ* is often used to refer to the site of action of any hormone, whether trophic or not (i.e., the prostate gland is as logically a target of androgens as the testis is a target of gonadotrophins).

The specificity of any hormone is a known fact. Hormones circulate in the bloodstream and reach cells in all regions of the body. We have no basic explanation, except for the receptor theory outlined

---

*The spelling of the hormones of the anterior pituitary has varied widely. Many investigators prefer to use the ending *tropic*, meaning "a turning," whereas others prefer the ending *trophic*, meaning "to nourish," signifying support of the fundamental metabolism of the involved cells. We prefer the latter ending, as the action of the pituitary hormones on specific end organs appears to be one of maintenance.

herein, for the observations that parathyroid hormone acts primarily on the bone and estrogens on the reproductive organs of the female, whereas thyroid hormones act on most cells. How response at the site of action is determined or modified by environmental or other factors is unknown. The specific makeup of the cells with regard to structure or biochemical function, which enables them to respond to one hormone but not another, is one of the most intriguing problems in endocrinology.

Despite the detailed lack of knowledge of the *site* of action of the hormones, many of the *mechanisms* of action are well documented. We know that the response of the target organ depends upon the amount of hormone present, i.e., a dose-response relationship exists. Second, a well-established mechanism of regulation is present—the effect of arterial blood sugar level on insulin secretion. With other organs such as the hypothalamus, the mechanisms are not so well understood, although much evidence suggests that some sort of controller balance exists.

The actions of the hormones can be summarized by saying that they act as catalysts and as such determine the *rates* of reaction rather than initiate *new* processes; they integrate activities between groups of cells; and they have relationships with other endocrine organs. Each of these processes will now be discussed in detail.

PROOF OF EXISTENCE OF A HORMONE

Despite the apparent wealth of information available, it is not always simple deciding whether a gland produces a hormone, what the hormone is, and what the hormone does. The classical proof for the existence of a hormone is in five steps.

1. *Extirpation.* The suspected organ is removed, and the effects of its removal on animals or tissues are noted, with particular reference to atrophy of organs, to metabolic defects, and to structural abnormalities.
2. *Replacement.* The suspected organ is transplanted, or, better still, an extract is made and injected into an animal from which the organ has been removed. The injected material should prevent the development of the changes noted on extirpation.
3. *Overdosage.* The extract of the suspected organ is given in large doses to normal animals, and to animals with the sus-

pected organ extirpated, to see if effects or overdosage can be demonstrated, and, perhaps, to demonstrate more clearly the effects of the endocrine material.
4. *Isolation.* The extract of the suspected organ is processed in an attempt to isolate a simple material that will yield the effects of the whole gland. This step should produce a single chemical entity that will reproduce all the effects of the gland as a whole. Sometimes, as in the case of the adrenal cortex, at least two substances are required to match effects obtained following injection of extracts of the entire gland. It is essential to identify the hormone actually secreted in response to proper stimulation as the substance isolated from the gland. Because extremely small amounts of material are usually added to a large volume of perfusing blood, this may be difficult. Chromatographic and electrophoretic procedures have been helpful, especially when combined with an appropriate type of isotopic labeling.
5. *Spontaneous defects.* It is usually possible to locate spontaneous defects of oversecretion and underproduction of the hormones and correlate them with specific organs in clinical cases.

It should be emphasized that the effects of the particular hormones in experimental animals cannot always be duplicated in the human being. Bovine and porcine growth-hormone preparations, for example, are active in many experimental animals but are inactive in humans, who respond only to primate preparations. In contrast, insulin, whatever its source, is highly effective in humans. For these and other reasons, the development of spontaneous defects is often the only method of detecting the hormone in a particular species.

OTHER CONSIDERATIONS

As a further complication to the study of endocrinology, the effects observed following hormone administration are often the results of interrelationships among the genetic composition of the test organism, the nervous system, the sensitivity of receptors, and the effects of one hormone upon the response to another. This can be illustrated by a simple example. The adrenal cortex is stimulated to produce its specific hormones by the adrenocorticotrophic hormone (ACTH) of the pituitary. The stimulus to the pituitary and thence to the gland is in part through nerve-mediated pathways via the hypothalamus, and all of these are further modified by genetic influence so that adrenals of various species produce different steroids under stimulation by the same ACTH preparation.

A further complication is the so-called permissive or enabling action of hormones. Some hormones—the adrenal cortical steroids in particular—appear to be necessary in certain small amounts in order for an organism to respond to various stimuli. This amount "permits" or enables the organism to respond to the stimulus. Increased amounts of hormone do not necessarily permit a greater response. In this sense, the permissive action is essentially a preparative one.

The hormones vary widely in composition (Table 1.1) and anatomical location. They range in size and complexity of structure from an aliphatic amine (epinephrine), through complex ring structures (steroids) and polypeptides (oxytocin, insulin), to proteins (chorionic gonadotrophin).

The hormones, which are elaborated by the pituitary, are all proteins although their sizes differ considerably. In addition, other secreting structures not under anterior pituitary control also produce

Table 1.1. The endocrine glands and their function.

Hormone	Principal Effects	Secreted by
Adrenocorticotropic hormone (ACTH)	Stimulates the adrenal cortex. Has less effect on aldosterone secretion than on other corticoids.	Pituitary
Thyrotropin (TSH)	Stimulates the thyroid gland.	Pituitary
Follicle-stimulating hormone (FSH)	Stimulates production of follicles by ovaries and spermatozoa by testes.	Pituitary
Luteinizing hormone (LH)	Causes follicle maturation and corpora lutea production in ovaries, or stimulates production of testosterone (male hormone) in testes.	Pituitary
Growth hormone (GH)	Governs normal growth and helps to regulate metabolism.	Pituitary
Prolactin (LTH)	Maintains corpora lutea, regulates milk production.	Pituitary
Antidiuretic hormone (ADH) or vasopressin	Regulates absorption of water in the kidney.	Neurohypophysis (part of the pituitary)
Oxytocin	Facilitates movement of sperm in fallopian tube, stimulates uterine muscle in childbirth, stimulates letdown of milk by breasts.	Neurohypophysis

Table 1.1. (Continued)

Hormone	Principal Effects	Secreted by
Cortisol and similar hormones	Regulates metabolism of sugar, protein, fat, minerals, and water.	Adrenal cortex (outer layer of adrenal gland)
Aldosterone and desoxycorticosterone	Regulate excretion and retention of minerals, particularly sodium and potassium by kidneys.	Adrenal cortex
Thyroid hormones, T_3 and T_4	Regulate rate of metabolism.	Thyroid
Estradiol 17-B	Regulates development of feminine characteristics and plays a part in ovulatory cycle.	Ovaries
Progesterone	Works with estrogen to regulate ovulation cycle and pregnancy.	Ovaries
Testosterone	Regulates development of male characteristics and reproductive system.	Testes
Insulin	Regulates utilization of sugar, proteins, and fats.	Pancreas (islets of Langerhans)
Glucagon	Helps to regulate utilization of sugar in opposition to insulin.	Pancreas (islets of Langerhans)
Parathyroid hormone (PTH)	Regulates calcium metabolism. Raises serum calcium.	Parathyroid glands
Thyrocalcitonin (TCT)	Helps to regulate calcium metabolism. Lowers serum calcium.	Thyroid
Adrenalin	Effects on brain and heart rate; mobilizes sugar and fat.	Adrenal medulla (inner layer of adrenal gland)
Noradrenaline	Increases force of heart contraction and constricts arterioles.	Adrenal medulla
Releasing factors	Individual ones cause release of ACTH, TSH, LH, FSH, prolactin, and growth hormone by pituitary. Individuals inhibit LH, FSH, ACTH, LTH, etc.	Brain (hypothalamus)
Somatostatin	Inhibits growth hormone, insulin, and glucagon production.	Hypothalamus
Somatomedin	Lays down collagen for bone under influence of GH.	Liver
MSH, melanocyte-stimulating hormone	Expansion of melanaphores.	Intermediate lobe of pituitary
Serotonin and melatonin	Regulates circadian cycles; light and dark responses. Reproductive processes.	Pineal
Prostaglandins	Have many effects on sex organs and other tissues.	Many areas of the body

hormones related to proteins (oxytocin, vasopressin, insulin, parathyroid hormone, chorionic gonadotrophin). The endocrines stimulated by the pituitary produce steroids or, in the case of the thyroid, the complex amino acid, thyroxine. The principal exception is the amine epinephrine, which is produced from the amino acid tyrosine by the adrenal medulla. This gland is not under control of the pituitary, but is a secreting homologue of the postganglionic cells of the autonomic nervous system.

SECRETION, TRANSPORT, AND EXCRETION

The endocrine glands have various methods of storing hormones within the glands until needed, when they release them into the bloodstream for transport to the site of action. For example, thyroid hormone is formed in the thyroid follicle as part of thyroglobulin complex and is hydrolyzed to be transported across the thyroid cells into the blood, where it is loosely combined with protein for transport in the blood. On the other hand, the polypeptide hormones are probably stored within the cell, either in discrete granules, as in the posterior pituitary, or in some unknown form. The steroid hormones may well be synthesized and released as needed, as high concentrations cannot be demonstrated in the glands. Endocrine secretion is designated as *merocrine* if the secretion takes place through the release of granules, and as *holocrine* if the entire cell breaks down to release the secretion.

The actual form in which a hormone may be secreted is not always known. The particular excretion form of a hormone found in the urine or the bile is often no indication of the actual active agent, because conjugation, degradation, and other alterations may have occurred between the secreting site and the site of action or after the secretion has fulfilled its function. Isolation of the hormone from the blood is more reliable but not always possible. The adrenal cortical steroids in the blood, for example, are about 70 percent glucuronide conjugated; yet, from the present evidence, it appears that these are inactive products on their way to excretion by the kidney, although peripheral hydrolysis may take place.

Since most hormones have a relatively short half-life ranging from minutes to hours, these substances must be rapidly inactivated. Proteins can be attacked by proteolytic enzymes and destroyed with no trace. The steroid hormones are conjugated with materials such as glucuronic acid or sulfate to make them more water-soluble and are then excreted in the urine, whereas other hormones are degraded by various other processes. Much of the research in endocrinology is devoted to determining the actual form of secretion of the hormones and the pathways of degradation. Since the advent of modern labeling techniques with radioisotopes, it has become easier to trace the hormones and to follow their pathways. Complications arise from the difficulty of establishing that an unusual label, such as I^{131} (radioactive iodine), on a protein molecule stays in position during the distribution of the injected hormone or as it acts on a target organ. It must always be kept in mind that the activity of any hormone is determined not only by the rate of synthesis, but also by the rate of degradation.

HORMONE ASSAY

The detection of hormones provides a serious problem for the biochemist and the endocrinologist. Some hormones are relatively simple to trace: the steroids can be analyzed chemically. The protein hormones offer a much more serious analytical problem. No less serious is the determination of such simple materials as thyroxine and epinephrine because of the extremely low levels present. Many sophisticated methods of chromatography, fluorescence, infrared analysis, mass spectroscopy, and the like have been applied to analysis of the endocrine molecules.

In some respects, the most sensitive and direct hormonal analysis is the bioassay, in which the response to varied dose levels of a particular hormone is measured in a suitably prepared animal through its effects on specific target organs. In fact, no chemical assay can be accepted until it has been correlated with an assay measuring the desired biological function. Under proper precautions and with extreme care, the bioassay technique is valuable, but many pitfalls lie in its use. Although it can be extremely sensitive, it may be very inaccurate since ranges of responses may easily vary by 100 percent or more. To be valid, an assay must be evaluated under a wide series of conditions. The response of animals varies with the number of doses of material (the same amount of material in twice the number of doses usually gives a larger response), the medium in which the hormone is administered, and many other factors unknown as well as unexpected.

The situation is further complicated because the response to a range of doses is usually not continuously proportional to the dose. As with most drugs, the relationship is such that a plot of the logarithm of the dose versus the response obtained gives a straight line (Figure 1.1) over a considerable range. Most animals fail to respond properly at either a high or a low dose so that an adequate range must be tested in order to locate a straight-line portion of the dose-response curve. Still other complications exist. Materials other than that under test may augment, decrease, or abolish the response. In biological extracts, unknown and unsuspected substances may interfere with the assay; this is especially true with assay of urine samples. A less obvious and usually neglected aspect is a chemical change in the test material after injection, producing an apparent response that may actually be only a secondary effect.

Any polypeptide or protein hormone sufficiently purified to give rise to a specific antibody can now be quantitated by an ingenious procedure originally devised by Berson and Yalow. An *in vitro* com-

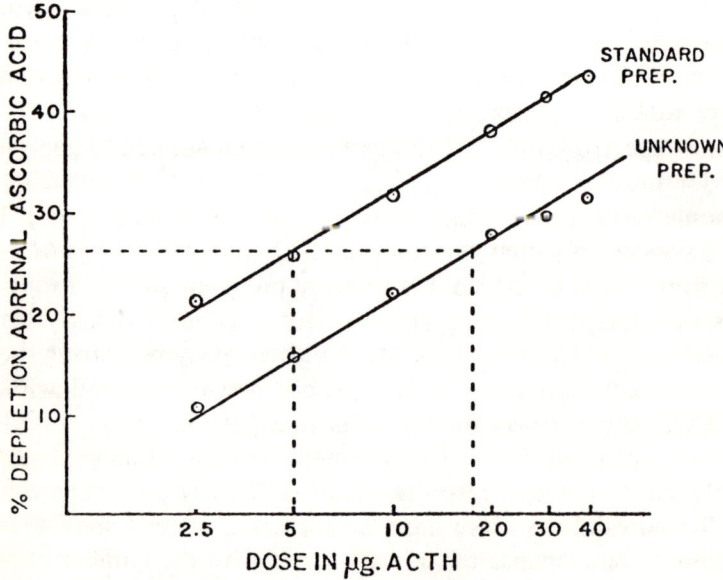

Figure 1.1. Assay of hormones. A dose-response curve for the effect of ACTH on the depletion of ascorbic acid in the adrenal gland.

plex of isotopically tagged (I^{131}) hormone plus its specific antibody is incubated with plasma containing unlabeled hormone. Because of competition for the limited amount of antibody present, some of the tagged hormone will be displaced from its binding with antibody and will be directly measured as a loss of antibody-bound radioactivity. This is known as the *immunochemical assay*. There will be further discussion of this topic later.

Assay of any type is complicated by the lack of good standards for comparison. There are international standards of many hormones, but most of these were prepared many years ago and, being extremely impure, are of low activity when compared to modern-day preparations. Many protein hormones now have been prepared 10 to 100 times as potent as the standard preparation. Materials that can be prepared in pure form, such as steroids, thyroxine, and epinephrine, can be compared directly on a weight basis rather than resorting to reference standards. Even in these instances, however, ambiguity can enter, as with the racemic form of an optically active material.

HOMEOKINESIS

All higher organisms are composed of cells of many types. These cells exist in a liquid medium, the *milieu interieur* of Claude Bernard. In order that the cells can perform their duties with maximum efficiency, it is necessary that the interstitial fluid environment be maintained constant in composition and that it be regularly exchanged so that nutrients can be added and waste products removed. The processes by which this occurs must operate continuously and with a high degree of sensitivity. The total sum of all the processes operating together to maintain constancy of environment for the cells was called *homeostasis*; however, we prefer the term *homeokinesis* to describe the sum of the dynamic processes acting to protect the cells of the body from undue change.

One of the major functions of the endocrine system is the maintenance of homeokinesis through such aspects as the regulation of osmotic concentration, salt concentration, and volume of the interstitial fluid. The entrance of material used for energy, the growth of the cells, and velocity of the enzymatic processes involved in the living cell are all under hormonal controls.

Although the endocrine system is a major component of the body's homeokinetic mechanisms, it is important to emphasize that the system must work in close conjunction with other mechanisms involving the whole organism. Regulation of salt concentration around cells would be of little importance if rate of blood flow, blood pressure, and vasoconstriction were also not adjusted to perfuse all organs at an optimum level and if the autonomic nervous system were not available to provide compensation for rapid changes in the environment of the organism as a whole.

Another important consideration enters the picture at this point. Each of the endocrine glands contributes its special function, but it must be remembered that homeokinesis is a process as a whole; this implies that any endocrine organ may have an effect on another in the overall control of cellular environment. This can be well demonstrated in many instances, but in many other cases the relationship is obscure. For example, the influence of the thyroid on general metabolism with consequent effects on the rate of production of other hormones is well known, while its relationship to growth hormone and insulin requirements in growth is not completely elucidated. The effects of other hormones on the parathyroids are virtually unknown.

Students in endocrinology should constantly keep in mind the principle of homeokinesis and the possible relationship of other parts of the whole organism to the endocrine system in their study of the individual gland.

THE FORM OF HORMONES

The hormones produced in specific endocrine glands appear in several forms in the body. The adrenal steroids are synthesized in the adrenal cortex and released into the bloodstream as active agents. On the other hand, many hormones are produced as *prohormones*, which means that they must be changed in form before they become active. Parathormone is released from the gland as a protein of MW 12,000 and then split into active moiety of MW 7,500 and an inactive residue. Insulin too is synthesized as a larger prohormone in three parts, the A-, B-, and C-chains. The C-chain is removed in the pancreatic cell before the active insulin—the A- and B-chains—are secreted. Still other hormones, particularly the thyroid hormones, are synthesized in an active form and then immediately placed in an inactive state through binding with protein. It is obvious that these mechanisms must be thoroughly understood before the actions of the hormones can be fully explained.

Many of the hormones are protein in nature. These hormones must be administered by injection rather than orally, and, as a result, they may cause the body to develop antibodies and foreign substances. As antibodies develop, the efficacy of the hormone diminishes. It has been known for many years that insulin may cause an antibody to develop. In some cases, the thyroid apparently leaks thyroglobulin into the bloodstream, and antibodies are formed to it, which may in time destroy the thyroid gland. Antihormones can be detected easily. The method can be illustrated by the following examples in which hormone is mixed with the plasma suspected of containing antibodies and then assayed in a biological system.

Test Substance	*Response (%)*
Hormone	100
Hormone + 1.0 ml plasma	10
Hormone + 0.5 ml plasma	40
Hormone + 0.25 ml plasma	80

The ability to form antibodies to protein hormones is the basis of the radioimmunoassay (RIA) mentioned previously.

2
Control Processes in Nature

All warm-blooded animals operate best in a constant cellular environment. This was appreciated by Claude Bernard when he outlined the *milieu interieur* theory and was expanded by Walter Cannon with his theory of control of milieu through the processes of homeostasis. Homeostasis or homeokinesis (see p. 11) are maintained through the control systems of the body.

An understanding of the control-system theory and its practice in physiology is essential to understanding the endocrine system and the feedback mechanisms that regulate secretion and metabolism.

The control systems of the body act by a process of negative feedback. In the regulation of blood sugar concentration, a high level of blood sugar in the extracellular fluid causes increased insulin secretion; this in turn causes decreased blood sugar concentration. In other words, the response is negative to the initiating stimulus (Figure 2.1). Conversely, if the blood sugar concentration falls too low, it causes feedback through the control system to decrease insulin secretion and allow blood sugar concentration to rise. This response also is in the opposite direction to the initiating stimulus.

In the aldosterone-sodium control mechanism, a high concentration of sodium ions causes decreased aldosterone secretion, which in turn diminishes sodium concentration. Thus, the response is negative to the elevated sodium level that initiates the response. Conversely, low

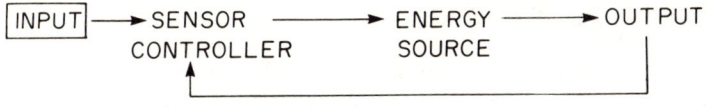

Figure 2.1. Feedback systems.

sodium concentration promotes increased aldosterone secretion and increased appetite for salt, both of which cause the sodium concentration to rise back toward normal. Thus, a low sodium level causes a higher level of aldosterone to ensue—again, a response that is negative to the initiating stimulus.

AMPLIFICATION, OR GAIN, OF A CONTROL SYSTEM

The degree of effectiveness with which a control system maintains constant conditions is called the amplification, or gain, of the system. For instance, let us assume that, for 24 hours, a person has been in a room where the temperature has been 60° F; suddenly, the temperature is increased to 110° F, a total increase of 50° F. However, the person's body temperature rises only from 98.0° to 99.0° F, because the human body automatically controls its own temperature within very narrow limits rather than following changes in atmospheric temperature. In this case, the change in atmospheric temperature is 49° F more than that in body temperature, which changes only 1° F. Therefore, we say that the gain of the control system is 49. In other words, for each degree change in body temperature that occurs, there would be 49 times as much additional change were it not for the control.

The majority of control systems of the body operate by negative rather than positive feedback. Positive feedback leads to instability and often death. Positive feedback is better known as a "vicious cycle," but actually a mild degree of positive feedback can be overcome by the negative-feedback control mechanisms of the body, so that a vicious cycle will fail to develop. In a few instances, particularly in the reproductive cycle, positive feedback is used to rapidly increase hormonal levels. The normal negative-feedback mechanisms for controlling the system can often overcome the positive feedback.

TRANSFER FUNCTIONS

Figure 2.2A through 2.2E illustrates easily understood properties of a control system. Figure 2.2F through 2.2H illustrates transfer functions that show a quantity x entering a block and a quantity y leaving the block. Each block means that y is related to x in accordance with the function that is placed inside the box.

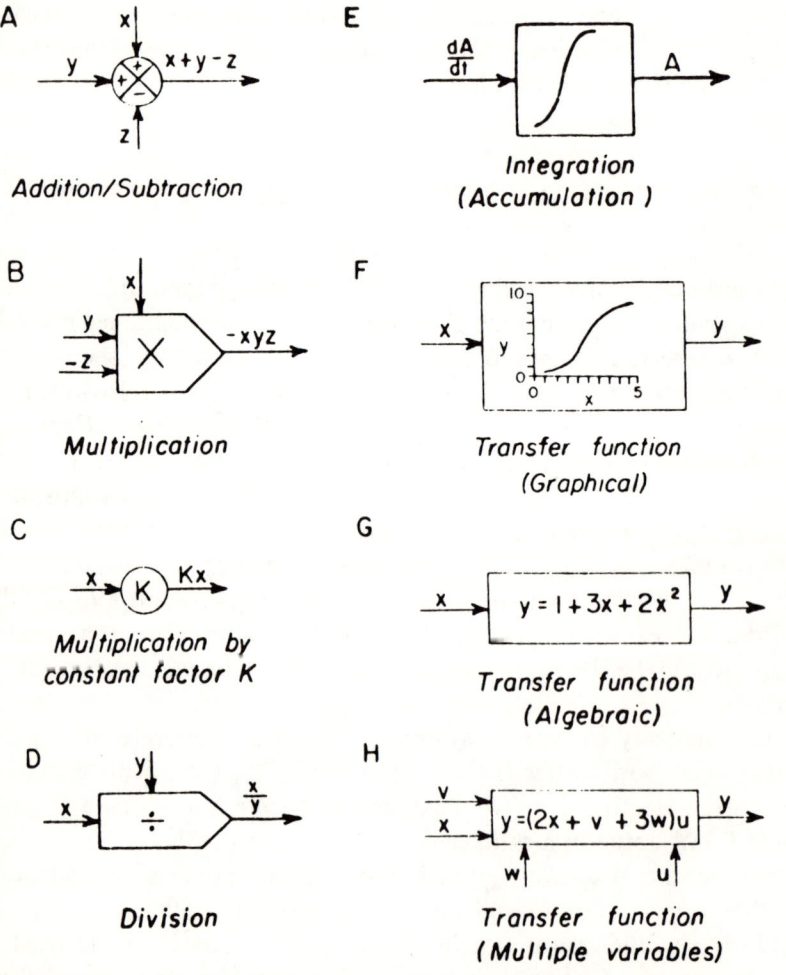

Figure 2.2. (A) through (H). Illustration of easily understood properties of a control system. ◀From A. C. Guyton, *Medical Physiology*, W. B. Saunders, Philadelphia, 1975, with permission.)

As an example, Figure 2.2F might represent the relationship between glucose concentration, s, in the extracellular fluids and the rate of insulin secretion, y, by the pancreas. This transfer function shows that when a low glucose concentration exists, essentially no insulin is secreted, but when there is a high concentration, very large quantities of insulin are secreted.

General Analysis of a Control System. Figure 2.1 illustrates a general analysis that can be applied to essentially any control system in the body. Note the box that is labeled *output*. This is the concentration, the rate, or the quantity that is to be controlled by the control system. The exact value of the controlled quantity is equal to the normal value of that quantity ± any disturbance that might try to change this value from the normal and ± the compensation of the control system.

More Complex Analysis of a Control System. Figure 2.3 illustrates an analysis of the control system for regulation of sodium concentration in the extracellular fluids. In this case, a person suddenly begins to drink concentrated salt solution at a continuous rate. Eventually, the sodium concentration in the person's extracellular fluids would increase 10 milliequivalents (meq)/liter if no compensation occurred for the increased rate of sodium intake. However, the increasing concentration of sodium in the extracellular fluids causes decreased

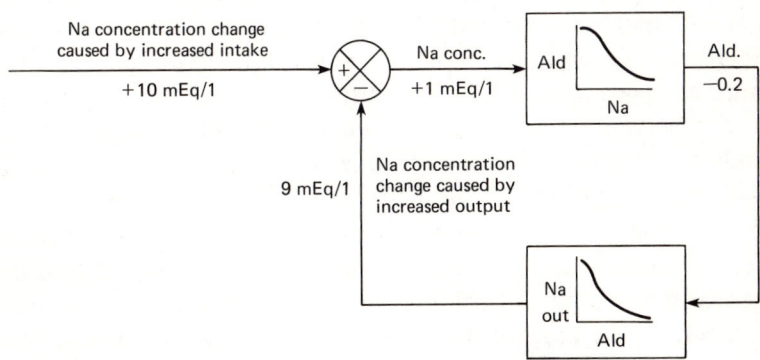

Figure 2.3. Analysis of a control system. The steady-state analysis of increased sodium intake on sodium concentration. (From A. C. Guyton, *Medical Physiology*, W. B. Saunders, Philadelphia, 1975, with permission.)

aldosterone concentration, which in turn causes increased output of sodium by the kidneys. This effect is sufficient to cause a decrease in sodium concentration of 9 meq/liter. Therefore, the large intake of sodium solution causes the sodium concentration in the body fluids to rise only 1 meq/liter.

Note that Figure 2.3 illustrates two transfer functions, one indicating the effect of sodium concentration on the aldosterone concentration and the other showing the effect of aldosterone concentration on the sodium concentration. Some control systems have 5, 10, or more steps, each of which can be represented by a transfer function.

Steady-State Versus Transient Analysis of Control Systems. The diagrams in Figures 2.1 and 2.3 represent steady-state analyses of two control systems. These analyses do not tell anything about the time courses of the changes; instead, they simply analyze what the condition will be after a complete state of equilibrium has developed. In some instances, the steady-state analyses are adequate to display the concepts of the different control systems of the body; more often, however, it is also important to know the time courses of changes in concentrations of different substances or changes in rates of activity. An analysis of a control system that can give the time courses of the changes is called a *transient analysis*.

Figure 2.4 illustrates a transient analysis of the same control system analyzed by the steady-state method in Figure 2.3. Here again, it is still the sodium concentration in the extracellular fluids that is being regulated, and the analysis shows what will happen to the sodium concentration when the rate of sodium intake or output from the body is equal to the rate of sodium intake minus the rate of sodium output through the kidney. In block 2 of Figure 2.4, the quantity of sodium in the body at any given time is the integral of the net rate of sodium intake or output. In block 3, the concentration of sodium in the body is equal to the quantity of sodium in the body divided by the volume of fluid (K_1) in which the sodium is distributed. In block 4, the rate of aldosterone secretion is a function of the sodium concentration. In block 5, the rate of aldosterone destruction is proportional to the aldosterone concentration in the body fluids. In block 6, the net rate of change of aldosterone in the body is equal to the rate of aldosterone secretion minus its rate of

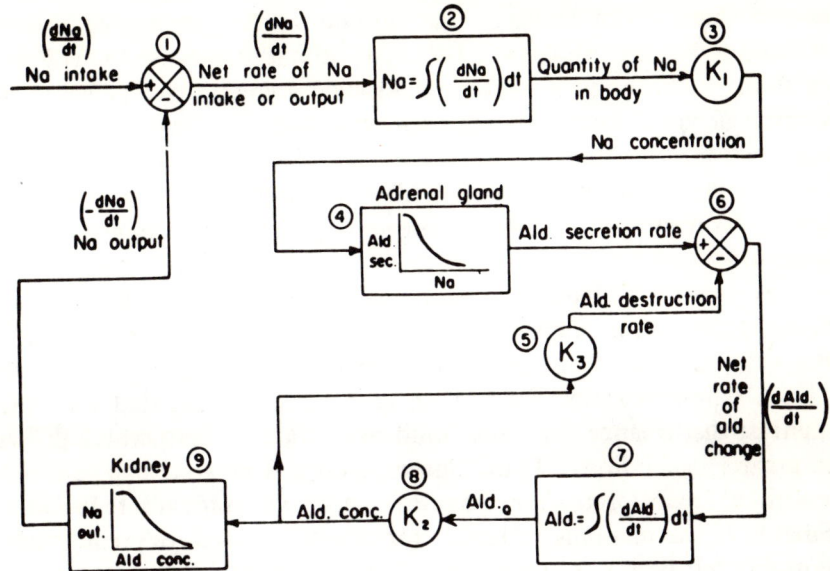

Figure 2.4. Regulation on sodium concentration. A transient analysis showing relationships between sodium concentration and various factors influencing it. (From A. C. Guyton, *Medical Physiology*, W. B. Saunders, Philadelphia, 1975, with permission.)

destruction. In block 7, the total quantity of aldosterone in the body at any give time is the integral of the net rate of aldosterone change in the body. In block 8, the aldosterone concentration is equal to the quantity of aldosterone multiplied by the reciprocal of the volume of fluid (K_2) in which it is distributed. In block 9, the rate of output of sodium by the kidney is a function of the aldosterone concentration. Thus, we have developed a closed-loop system in which a series of complex reactions cause a feedback that prevents the sodium concentration in the body fluids from changing significantly even though the sodium intake increases or decreases drastically.

OSCILLATION OF CONTROL SYSTEMS

Unfortunately, even negative-feedback control systems sometimes become unstable and oscillate. The reason for lack of oscillation in most control systems of the body is that almost all control systems are highly damped as a result of the basic organization of the control system itself. For instance, the sodium control system of Figure 2.3 and 2.4 does not show oscillation, primarily because the volume of fluid in the body is so large that even a greatly changed rate of sodium accumulation requires many hours to significantly alter the sodium concentration. In the meantime, the other parts of the control system can adapt themselves almost completely to the changing sodium concentration, thereby preventing any overresponse of the system.

It is possible to have increasing oscillation, driving oscillation, and damped oscillation, depending on whether the amplitude increases, stays the same, or decreases. In the first case, the system is said to have a damping ratio of less than zero, which means that even the slightest disturbance can cause mild oscillation at first, which grows to greater oscillations. If the damping ratio is greater than zero but less than 1, any oscillation that does occur will gradually fade away. Finally, if the damping ratio is 1 (critically damped) or greater than 1, there will be no oscillation at all; instead, sudden changes, such as the sudden increase in sodium intake in the analysis of Figure 2.4, will simply cause slow change, with the system gradually approaching a new state of equilibrium.

A few control systems, such as the one that causes the monthly sexual cycle of the female, continue to oscillate indefinitely.

A more technical explanation of control theory is included in the appendix, and oscillating systems are discussed in more detail in the section on biorhythms.

RHYTHMS IN BIOLOGICAL ACTIVITY

The control processes in biological systems are very similar to those in physical systems. As mentioned previously, control systems, particularly those that are biological in origin, have set points (e.g., blood sugar level, blood sodium concentration), and the feedback is designed to operate with a reasonably small error around such points. Sometimes, the set point appears to be highly variable, i.e., the response of various accessory sex organs to hormones varies widely with the point in the menstrual cycle at which they are measured.

The very phenomenon of feedback promotes oscillation. As the signal hunts around the set point for optimum response, a sinusoidal form of response is generated. It has already been pointed out that if the feedback to the system reinforces the oscillation, or occurs in phase with it, the feedback is positive and augments the signal. This creates an inherently unstable system.

Negative feedback results in damping and a gradually diminishing error signal. Oscillations in a system generally arise from several sources, all of which are present in a biological system. Oscillation may be harmonic and occur regularly and at constant amplitude. A sequence of all-or-no responses in a repetitive mode such as nerve responses may appear to be an oscillatory phenomenon and unrelated transients in a system may induce oscillations that obscure the basic physiological mechanisms.

In a biological system, the oscillations are not always clearly defined. Many of the systems are balanced by large energy reservoirs, which tend to decrease system fluctuations, and the system may therefore be highly damped. The damping may be altered by time lag; high gain, which promotes instability; dead space, which decreases sensitivity; hysteresis, which does not return the system to its original state; and information lack in the feedback channel.

The relationship of the preceding, more or less theoretical background to endocrinology becomes clear when we consider the many examples of oscillation that are readily apparent in the endocrine system. The monthly cycle of the female is an obvious example, and dozens of other examples can be cited.

Any oscillations must arise first in the cell and be coupled to the enzyme systems. Many years ago, Britton Chance demonstrated that the enzyme systems concerned with carbohydrate metabolism exhibited oscillatory phenomena and that the speed and amplitude of oscillation could be changed with environmental factors. Furthermore, these systems were self-damping, as they should be in order to prevent runaway phenomena. The coupling between oscillators, which allows the enzymatic system to determine the rate of an overall process, is not well understood.

A Bode plot (Figure 2.5) of gain against frequency indicates that an oscillating system should have an optimum-frequency response. We do not know the characteristics of many biological oscillators so we cannot predict optimum frequencies. It is interesting that many biological phenomena do operate on a precisely timed schedule, ranging in frequency from seconds to months and perhaps to years.

The oscillations, as they are correctly called in an engineering sense,

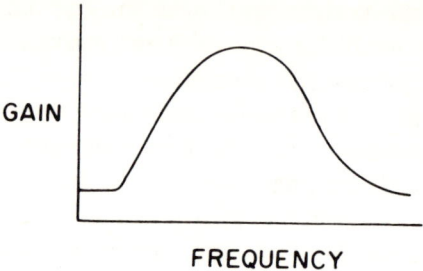

Figure 2.5. Bode plot of control system.

have long been recognized by biologists and lumped under the terms *physiological clock, circadian rhythms,* or *biological rhythms*. Biologists have known for years of circadian rhythms (varying with time), diurnal rhythms (varying with time of day), photoperiodic rhythm (varying with light or dark), and biochemical rhythms.

Long before the precise mechanism of hypothalamic and pituitary interactions were known, it had been established that ACTH had a distinct diurnal rhythm and that the release of corticoids by the adrenal paralleled the release of ACTH, although out of phase by some hours. Biologists have observed the seasonal development of accessory sex organs in most domestic and tame animals, and the annual migration of birds is a well-known fact. Although the maintenance of homeostasis and reproduction are distinctly hormonal influences, the actual effect of hormones as opposed to other nervous inputs has not been well established. With the development of modern radioimmunoassay techniques, it has become relatively easy to track rhythmic changes in hormone concentration. In the following discussion, we will look at some of the endocrine rhythms. It should be clear, however, that in most cases we do not understand the set point or the oscillatory phenomena.

One of the clear-cut rhythms is that of the growth hormone, which appears in the blood of all persons at all ages. It is present in extremely low concentrations during most of the day. However, a sharp peak lasting only a short time occurs in almost all normal people about 45 minutes after entering a deep sleep (or rapid eye movement, REM, sleep). The feedback for growth hormone is unknown, and therefore the purpose of the rise is pure speculation. It cannot be well correlated with the only parameter that is known to be directly connected to growth-hormone concentration changes—the blood sugar. As growth hormone is related to growth and repair, it has been suggested that, as metabolism and bodily demands slow in sleep, the secretion of growth hormone then triggers repair and cell-replacement mechanisms. In the case of overstimulation of the pituitary with overproduction of growth hormone, however, the diurnal rise does not occur.

Other hormones follow obscure patterns. Prolactin (LTH) apparently serves no function in most mammals except for maintenance of the corpus luteum during the latter phases of the estrous or menstrual cycle. Yet, LTH is secreted regularly on a daily basis, with a peak at 4 p.m. There is no detectable relationship between time, concentration of hormone, or phase of the cycle. It is possible to presume that a daily secretion occurs but that no effect is produced until a target organ with the correct receptors arises and can respond. Nevertheless, this offers no explanation of *why* the diurnal variation occurs.

Many wild and domestic animals have dramatic increases in testes weight and spermatogenesis in the spring. Both of these are related to the secretion of luteinizing hormone (LH) and androgen production. A change in androgen production or in sensitivity of the target organs must occur.

Biological rhythms may be superimposed on each other. In androgen production, for example, there is a daily variation that is imposed upon a seasonal variation.

It is possible to speculate that this is caused by nervous or other impulses, which "turn on" the pituitary, causing the subsequent secretion of its hormones. Although almost all hormones have a diurnal variation, the peaks of secretion occur at different times, indicating different control systems. In many cases, the change in hormone concentration is 10 times the base level so that chance variation is not likely. This diurnal variation without a known feedback suggests that this phenomenon may be a "forced" rhythm or oscillator set at a given speed by another oscillator coupled to it.

As F. E. Yates pointed out, this coupling is difficult to decipher. In the ultimate, all reaction depends on enzymatic chemical action in a time domain of milliseconds, whereas the same set of reactions examined at the glandular level does not reveal any of the fast kinetic reactions but shows an overall reaction rate of minutes to hours.

Nevertheless, the unseen reactions are coupled to the longer phases and must drive them in some fashion. Yates also emphasized that the reaction may be a *rate*-sensitive rather than a *mass*-sensitive function. Because many other reactions are also going on in the body and may contribute metabolites or rate changes, which are noise to the information system under test, it is difficult to determine the parameters.

The cyclic sexual phenomenon has already been mentioned several times. The precise timing of estrogen, follicle-stimulating hormone (FSH), and LH secretions in sequence is necessary for a normal menstrual cycle to occur. One of the more apparent aspects of the sexual cycle is the release of prolactin, which appears to be necessary to maintain the corpus luteum after its formation. Prolactin has a diurnal variation and apparently serves as its own feedback. In addition to the monthly cycle of gonadotrophins in women (which does not occur in men), there are longer rhythms related to age and development. The drug clomiphene will release gonadotrophins in the normal adult, but will not stimulate the pituitary in the prepuberal child. This lack of response may be due to receptor sensitivity. Such a change in sensitivity can easily be demonstrated in women who are pretreated with estrogen. Luteinizing-hormone releasing factor (LRF) in the same dose causes a threefold greater release of gonadotrophins but does not change the diurnal variation of a peak at 3 a.m. and low at 2 p.m.

The relationship between LTH and corticoids can be tied to another relationship—that of body weight. LTH causes either deposition of fat in adipose tissue or the release of nonesterified fatty acids (NEFA) depending on its relationship to corticoid secretion. As corticoids also have an influence on fat metabolism, it is easy to suppose either an additive or subtractive function. As Table 2.1 clearly shows, there is a distinct relationship between the diurnal variation in LTH and corticoids, and the presence or absence of obesity. The phase angle between the two secretions appears to be the determining factor, and it is probable that this in turn may be conditioned by the solution of corticoids in fat and the resulting maintenance of high levels.

Unfortunately, these interesting data do not give us a complete picture of oscillatory phenomena in the endocrine system. We do not usually know the phase shifts between one secretion and the

Table. 2.1. The relationship between the peak of LTH secretion and corticoids secretion illustrating a constant phase shift.

State	Time of LTH Peak Secretion	Time of Corticol Peak Secretion
Normal	3 p.m.	6 a.m.
Lean	12 midnight	6 a.m.
Fat	6 p.m.	6 a.m.

subsequent action. ACTH is maximally secreted at 6 a.m., which is followed by a peak corticoid excretion at 2 p.m. We do not know if this 8-hour delay is usual, if it is the same in most species, or how it can be changed by circumstances. LTH has a diurnal variation with a monthly rhythm imposed upon it; in domestic animals, a seasonal variation is also imposed. The relationship between these is not clear, and we do not know if phase shifts (such as that discussed between LTH and cortisol) would modify the picture.

TRF (thyrotrophin-releasing factor) secretion and therefore thyroid secretion are modified by cortisol levels. Cortisol usually peaks in the human plasma at about 6 a.m. TRF secretion begins after sleep at 12 p.m. and falls immediately when the morning cortisol peak occurs. Cortisol secretion is a true diurnal phenomenon conditioned by sleep. The peak at 6 a.m. persists in the blind, indicating that light and dark play no part. Changes in the sleep pattern will change the peak hormone production by a corresponding amount.

Some of the relationships in the endocrine system are determined by the secretions of two hormones that produce opposite effects on the same control system. The relationship of calcitonin and parathyroid hormone (PTH) and of insulin and glucagon come instantly to mind. This relationship provides a point of control that does not require a set point for either variable. Riggs has defined the accuracy of this kind of regulation as the *homeostatic index.*

Another interesting system that oscillates is the secretion of antidiuretic hormone (ADH) in the control of body water (Figure 2.6). E. M. Reeves and A. C. Guyton have shown that the oscillations are controlled by water content of the body, which is in turn a function of water absorbed from gut (turnoff) and water intake into the stom-

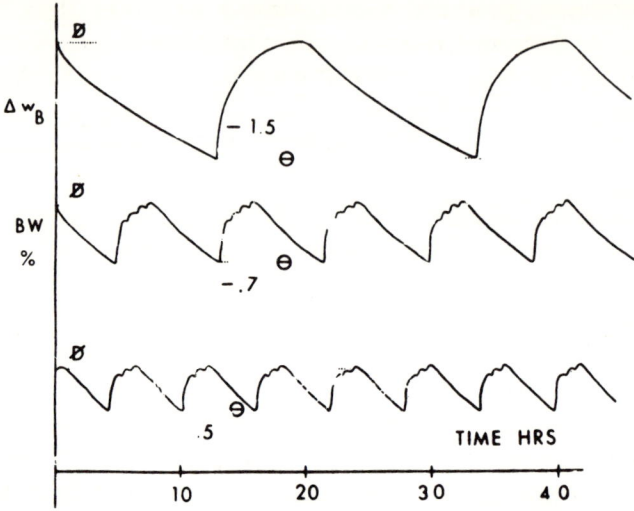

Figure 2.6. The effect on body water of drinking. The diagram illustrates the cyclic changes in body water with time. Body water is held constant and drinking threshold varied. (From Reeve, E. M. and A. C. Guyton, *Physiological Basis of Circulatory Transport*, W. B. Saunders, Philadelphia, 1963, with permission.)

ach (turn-on). There are set points both for drinking and for urinary shutdown. If these are too close, both are reduced; if they are too far apart, something like diabetes insipidus may result.

The study of the secretion of cortisone has been an interesting example in control theory because, in one case study, the dynamics have lead to prediction of an unknown metabolic pathway, later confirmed by chemical analysis.

REMARKS ON CONTROL IN THE ENDOCRINE SYSTEM

As each gland is discussed, its control system will also be discussed. It has been mentioned that feedback is important in the control of endocrine secretion. In many cases, it is impossible to determine where the feedback actually occurs. When the hypothalamus secretes a releasing factor, which in turn causes output of a trophin from the pituitary, which in turn increases the production of a target organ, there are many sources of feedback. The end-organ hormone may feedback to the hypothalamus; it is possible for a hormone to serve as its own feedback to the producing cells. In other cases, the control of hormone production is governed by other than hormone feedback. Aldosterone is apparently controlled by the sodium concentration in the plasma, and the parathyroids by the calcium concentration. The control of insulin by the blood sugar level is not so clear-cut because the feedback may actually be a metabolic product rather than a glucose concentration itself. Feedback may also be through nervous channels. The control of ADH by osmoreceptors and of aldosterone by hypothetical volume receptors are cases in point. Growth hormone (GH) is a notable example of where the feedback mechanisms are unknown.

The feedback may be modified by physical factors in addition to the humoral factors and secretion rate. Generally, the hormone must be free to enter cells or bind to cell plasma membranes before it can become active. If the hormone is bound in the plasma, activity can be greatly altered. The difference in activity of triiodothyronine and tetraiodothyronine can be traced in large part to the tenfold difference in binding to plasma protein. The influence of number and presence of receptors on hormone activity has already been mentioned.

Any attempt to explain the dynamics of hormone action must take these factors into account. When we consider that many of these ideas have come into prominence in the last few years, it is clear that we may expect much new progress in understanding endocrine dynamics in the near future.

References

Aschoff, J. *Circadian Clocks*. Amsterdam: Elsevier, 1865.
Bunning, E. *Physiological Clock*. London: Oxford University Press, 1973.
Clark, R. H. and B. L. Baker. "Circadian Periodicity in Concentration of Prolactin in Rat Hypophysis." *Science* **143** (1964): 373.
Franchimont, P. and H. Burger. *HGH and Gonadotrophins in Health and Disease*. Amsterdam: North Holland Publishing, 1975.
Gual, C. and E. Rosenberg. *Hypothalamic Hypophysio-trophic Hormones*, Amsterdam: Excertpa Medica, 1973.
Hague, E. B. "Photo-Neuro-Endocrine Effects in Circadian Rhythms." *Annals of the New York Academy of Science* **117** (1964):1.
Halberg, F., J. H. Galicich, F. Ungar, and L. A. French. "Circadian ACTH Activity." *Proc. Soc. Exp. Biol. & Med.* **118** (1965):414.
Pasteel, J. L. and F. J. G. Ebling. *Human Prolactin*. Amsterdam: Excerpta Medica, 1973.

Reeves, E. M. and A. C. Guyton. *Physical Basis of Circulatory Transport.* Philadelphia: W. B. Saunders, 1976.
Riggs, D. S. *Mathematical Approach to Physiological Problems.* Baltimore: Williams & Wilkins, 1963.
Sollberger, A. *Biological Rhythm Research.* Amsterdam: Elsevier, 1965.
Yates, F. E. "Systems Analysis in Biology." In Brown, J. H. U., *Biomedical Engineering.* Philadelphia: F. A. Davis, 1971.

3
The Cellular Activity of Hormones

It is a *sine qua non* in biological activity that substances must reach the cell on which they act. This simplistic statement is often difficult to demonstrate where hormones are concerned because the mechanisms of hormone action are not always well understood and are so varied in nature.

The examination of the products of an endocrine gland and of an assay of blood or plasma for the products can be misleading as to the active substances. The gland may contain many precursors that have not yet been synthesized into the hormone; it may contain prohormones that are inactive. The blood may contain not only the active hormone but prohormones. It almost always contains products of hormone degradation, which may be on the way to excretion or destruction by the liver or kidney. The best example is the adrenal cortex. Cortisol and aldosterone are accepted as *the* active adrenal steroids in the human, yet dozens of steroids are found in the adrenal gland, the blood, and the urine.

The problem of activity is further complicated by the many ways in which the tissues handle hormones. Some hormones appear to exert their effects and are then released from the site of action essentially unchanged. The action of estrogen on the uterus appears to be a matter of time of contact, rather than of any change in the estrogen. On the other hand, cortisone is rapidly destroyed in the tissues.

In at least one other case, the hormone secreted by the gland (testosterone by the testes) must be converted by tissue metabolism to another substance (dihydrotestosterone) before it can become active on the accessory sex organs. It does appear that any hormone activity must depend on the preferential retention of the hormone by the target organ. This implies the presence of a substance—a receptor—specifically for the hormone, and located only in the target organs.

SITE OF ACTION OF THE HORMONES

The specificity of hormone action may be determined by the location of the receptors. This may explain why some hormones somatotrophic corticoids, insulin, thyroid) act on most cells, whereas other hormones (sex hormones) act only on specific target organs. The hypothalamic and pituitary hormones appear to be rather specific, yet certain interrelationships suggest that even here the targeting is not totally specific.

It is a well-accepted idea that hormonal ultimate action must be in the synthesis of protein and hence in the enzymes, which produce the chemical-reaction-rate changes that are finally revealed as the hormonal cellular action. In some way, the hormone (except for a few specific examples, such as insulin) must be able to influence the nucleus and stimulate DNA to the production of genetic codes, which are transmitted to ribosome and transfer RNA. The ribosome is then able to synthesize new enzymes in a specific way to perform the desired activity. The site of activity of the hormone can be clearly demonstrated by blocking protein synthesis or by stimulating it. As we will see later, it is also possible to block the pathway by which the hormone reaches the nuclear mechanisms. Table 3.1 gives an indication of our present understanding of blocking agents.

Table 3.1. Inhibitors of protein synthesis.

Inhibitor	Site of Action
Actimyosin D	RNA synthesis
Hydroxyurea	DNA synthesis
Puromycin	Translation
Caffeine	Cyclic AMP stimulation
Imidazol	Cyclic AMP inhibition
Ouabain	Sodium transport

The mechanisms by which the hormone exerts its influence on the cell's synthetic processes are just now becoming clear. Two different pathways must be utilized, depending upon the hormone. In one path, the hormone can penetrate the cell wall and reach the cytoplasm or the nucleus. Hormones that can enter the cell (such as thyroxine) must be of a small size and the proper molecular structure. On the other hand, the protein hormones cannot penetrate the cell and must exert their influence through secondary mechanisms.

The best example of a hormone of the first type (the *first messenger* theory) is estrogen. Estrogen readily penetrates the cell wall of its target organs and is bound in the nucleus. Estrogen is bound to specific *receptors*, and few nonestrogens are bound to estrogen receptors. The estrogen receptors are dimeric proteins with a molecular weight of 222,000.

When estrogen penetrates the cell, it is first bound to cytoplasmic receptors. It is then "activated" and transported to the nucleus where it initiates specific DNA processes. The formation of the nuclear receptor complex is absolutely dependent on the estrogen-cytosol complex to complete the formation. This then leads to increased RNA synthesis.

Those hormones that cannot penetrate the cell to initiate processes directly must either act at the cell membrane or through some other process using a *second messenger* system.

The hormones insulin and vasopressin (ADH) apparently operate largely by altering the permeability of the cell membrane to glucose and water, respectively. The protein hormones and epinephrine at the beta receptor must act through a second messenger in order to stimulate protein synthesis. It is apparent that the receptors for these hormones are located in the cell membrane and that, when the receptor-hormone complex is formed, the activated molecule is able to trigger the release of cyclic AMP (c-AMP) through the release of adenyl cyclase or some other substance in the cell membrane (Figure 3.1). The present theory than assumes that c-AMP is able to trigger the many protein synthetic processes.

Although it is clear that c-AMP is involved in the process, the mechanisms are not at all clear. The use of drugs that either block or stimulate the release of c-AMP have profound effects on the extent of hormone action. Furthermore, c-AMP has been involved in the activity of many hormones (Table 3.2). Despite the evidence, it is

Table 3.2. Some hormone actions mediated by changes in cyclic AMP.

Hormone	Tissue	Effect
	Increased Cyclic AMP Levels	
Adrenocorticotrophic hormone	Adrenal cortex	↑ Steroidogenesis
	Fat (rat)	↑ Lipolysis
Luteinizing hormone	Corpus luteum, ovary, testis	↑ Steroidogenesis
	Fat	↑ Lipolysis
Catecholamines	Fat	↑ Lipolysis
	Liver	↑ Glycogenolysis, ↑ gluconeogenesis
	Skeletal muscle	↑ Glycogenolysis
	Heart	↑ Inotrophic effect
	Salivary gland	↑ Amylase secretion
	Uterus	Relaxation
Glucagon	Liver	↑ Glycogenolysis, ↑ gluconeogensis, ↑ induction of enzymes
	Fat	↑ Lipolysis
	Pancreatic alpha cells	↑ Insulin release
	Heart	↑ Isotropic effect
Thyroid-stimulating hormone	Thyroid	↑ Thyroid hormone release
	Fat	↑ Lipolysis
Melanocyte-stimulating hormone	Dorsal frog skin	↑ Darkening
Parathyroid hormone	Kidney	↑ Phosphaturia
	Bone	↑ Ca^{+2} resorption
Vasopressin	Toad bladder, renal medulla	↑ Permeability
Hypothalamic releasing factors	Adenohypophysis	↑ Release of trophic hormones
Prostaglandins	Platelets	↓ Aggregation
	Thyroid	↑ Thyroid hormone release
	Adenohypophysis	↑ Release of trophic hormones
	Decreased Cyclic AMP Levels	
Insulin	Fat	↓ Lipolysis
	Liver	↓ Glycogenolysis, ↓ gluconeogenesis
Prostaglandins	Fat	↓ Lipolysis
	Toad bladder	↓ Permeability
Catecholamines (β-adrenergic stimuli)	Frog skin	↓ Darkening
	Pancreas	↓ Insulin release
	Platelets	↓ Aggregation
Melatonin	Frog skin	↓ Darkening

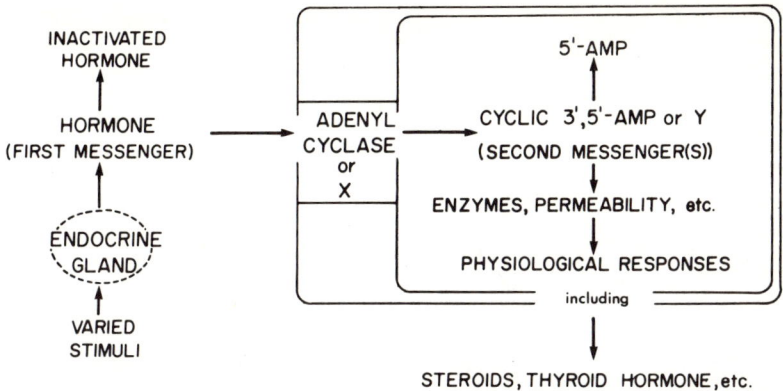

Figure 3.1. The second-messenger theory.

not at all clear how a single simple substance c-AMP is able to trigger DNA to perform a variety of synthetic processes, varying from one hormone to another. A more attractive theory is that c-AMP serves as a cofactor to trigger or activate cytoplasmic receptors, each a different protein for each hormone, which then in turn are able to turn on the genetic mechanism.

THE ROLE OF RECEPTORS

The existence of protein cellular receptors for hormones, although newly discovered is already a vital part of endocrinology. Many hormone actions can now be explained on the basis of receptor theory. Many of the hormone antagonists—drugs that block or alter endocrine function—can also be explained on this basis. Spiralactone, which blocks the action of aldosterone and competes with the steroid for binding sites on the kidney tubules, operates in this fashion. Alteration of the structure of the steroids (for example, addition of a methoxy group to estrogens) will prevent binding to the accessory sex-organ tissues while other properties are retained.

Hormones that are similar in structure may compete for binding sites. The weak salt-retaining properties of progesterone may be due to competition with cortisol for binding sites in the kidney. Figure 3.2 illustrates the widely differing activity of two estrogens in the same system, which may be a function of receptor-binding. Occa-

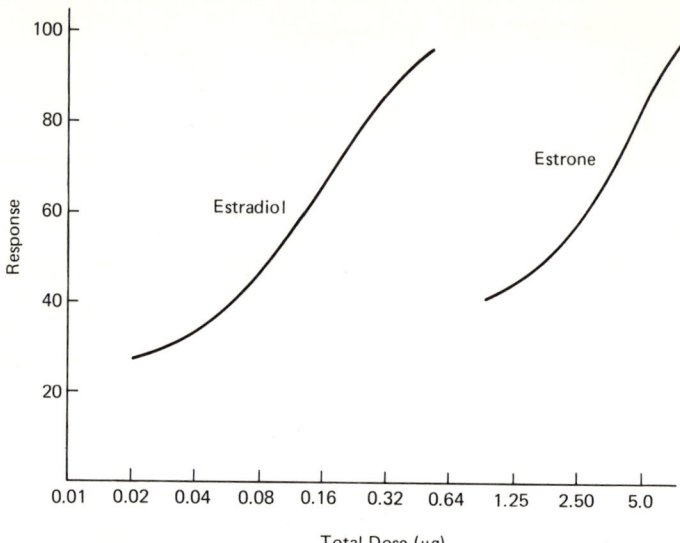

Figure 3.2. The activity of two estrogens on the same system. This may be a reflection of receptor activity.

sionally, the binding sites or the receptors may be missing altogether as a result of a genetic mishap. When this happens with androgen-binding sites in the male, feminization results, because the androgens cannot produce the normal effect. The salt-losing syndrome in Eskimo children may also be due to a lack of aldosterone receptors.

The number of receptors is not constant. Estrogen administration leads to the production of more receptors, whereas deprivation results in a decrease in numbers. The increase in receptors when steroid is administered can be blocked with RNA synthesis-blocking agents indicating the genetic relationship. There may well be a physiological basis for a change in receptor numbers. Changes in progesterone concentration during the menstrual cycle are closely paralleled by a change in the number of uterine receptors, which may reflect changes in sensitivity to the hormone.

The work of McGuire et al. suggests that development of cancer of the breast may parallel estrogen-receptor concentration in breast tissue, as breast cancer is hormone-dependent; this finding may be of great significance.

ASSAY OF RECEPTORS

The development of the radioimmunoassay (RIA) technique lead to an order-of-magnitude increase in sensitivity of hormone assays. A short discussion of the technique and its application is in order here because receptors are measured by the method, as are most protein hormones.

The technique is relatively simple in process but requires infinite care to obtain consistent results. An antibody is prepared to any desired substance by injection into a recipient of a different genetic strain (e.g., horse, rabbit). If the substance tested is not capable of causing an immune response because it is nonantigenic (steroids, for example), the chemical is complexed with an antigenic protein and an antibody is formed to the complex. The antibody is purified for analysis.

To conduct an analysis, the antibody is saturated with a radioactive labeled antigen until all sites are occupied. The known samples, containing a known amount of antigen with a measured radioactivity, are now mixed with the unknown sample to be tested. An equilibrium rate reaction occurs, and an exchange of unknown sample with known labeled antigen occurs. The amount of exchange is directly related to the ratio of the concentrations of the two antigens. The activity decreases in direct proportion to the amount of unknown sample present. For example, if the known and unknown were in *equal* concentration, the radioactivity would be one-half or 50 percent, of the original. The basic process can be modified to increase the sensitivity. Another *second* antibody can be made to the *first* antibody and used to precipitate it, after it is combined with the unknown to increase selectivity. By this technique, it has been possible to determine that the average cell contains about 11,000 insulin receptors. In this case, of course, antibodies were made to the isolated receptor protein, and the binding was determined. The accuracy of the binding to the desired protein is not always totally satisfactory.

It is also possible to tag hormones with radioactive atoms, and by radioautography to determine cellular location of binding and degree of binding. This technique will obviously not measure the number of sites.

The activity of a hormone is a function of its intrinsic activity or its affinity for receptors. Binding of a hormone to a receptor follows a simple law of mass action. Two phenomena must be taken into account. First, the hormones must be absorbed on the surface of the protein receptors, which follows the absorption law (Langmuir equation). Second, it must combine with the receptor (enzyme-substrate relationship) as defined by the Michaelis-Menten equations.

The intrinsic activity of the hormone is inversely proportional to the number of receptors that must be occupied to produce a response. In other words, the more active the hormone, the fewer the sites that may be occupied in order to produce a response. There are both high-affinity, low-capacity, and high-capacity, low-affinity hormone-binding sites, which vary with the hormone. It may be that the competitive relationship between hormone antagonists may be due to affinity change with alteration in structure.

HORMONAL INTERRELATIONSHIPS

Throughout this book, we will attempt to illustrate the close-knit ties between the endocrine organs and metabolic processes. The antagonistic action of PTH and thyrocalcitonin, and of insulin and glucagon will be mentioned. The effect of adrenocortical steroids and insulin on blood sugar will be discussed, as will other similar relationships.

In order to present a cohesive picture of metabolic processes, we will now summarize these interrelationships in the control of metabolism.

The most important of the metabolic controls are those that regulate blood sugar because such regulation may require anabolism or catabolism of proteins and fats as well as carbohydrates in order to maintain the desired level of control. Figure 3.3 serves to illustrate

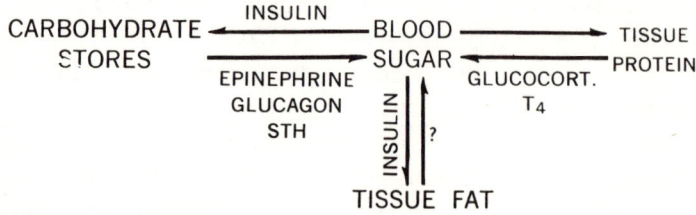

Figure 3.3. An illustration of some interrelationships among various hormones in the regulation of intermediary metabolism, particularly emphasizing the central position of the blood sugar. Formation of new body protein is not considered here.

this point. The influence of several hormones on both anabolic and catabolic processes is clearly demonstrated in the regulation of blood glucose.

The model can be extended to include other processes and to indicate the complexity of regulation as shown in Figure 3.4. Here, information relating to physiological use, hunger, and excretion have been added to the model together with sites of activity and the interrelationships of various controls.

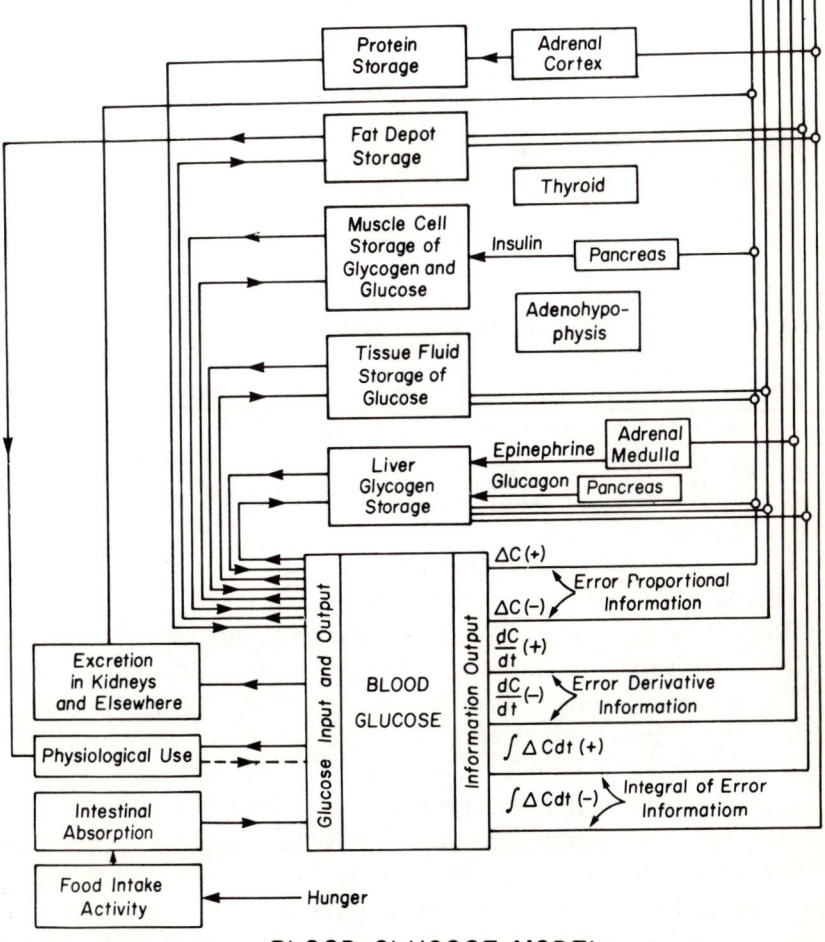

BLOOD GLUCOSE MODEL

Figure 3.4. The influence of many factors on the overall control of blood glucose. (Taken from Stear and Kadish, *Hormonal Control System*, American Elsevier, New York, 1954).

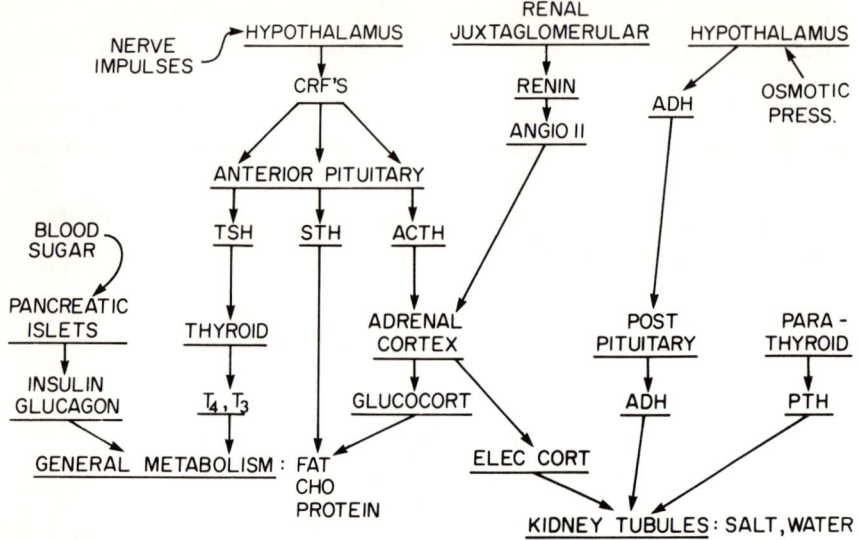

Figure 3.5. An illustrative example of the complex interrelationships of various endocrine organs on the control of metabolism.

It must be kept in mind that the endocrine glands do not operate alone and that endocrine processes are controlled in turn by the nervous system and by other processes that determine circadian rhythms. Figure 3.5 shows the relationship between general metabolism and salt and water metabolism, which is intimately tied into the overall body processes, as will be shown later.

The metabolic processes influenced by hormones are summarized in Table 3.3. Here, the wide variety of activity and the often contradictory effect that serves as a counterbalance are clearly shown.

The control of metabolism by the endocrine system operates in three ways. First, the action of the endocrine glands may be antagonistic and serve as a counterbalance. This is particularly true where it is essential for life that the processes be controlled within narrow limits such as the blood sugar and plasma calcium levels. Next, the effects of the hormones may be additive (for example, the effects of glucagon and epinephrine in raising the blood sugar). This type of response may serve to provide rapidly increased supplies of glucose for emergencies. Finally, some hormones may be "permissive"; that is, they permit the effects of other hormones to occur when the permis-

Table 3.3. The effect on endocrines and metabolism.

Hormone	Effect on Fat Metabolism	Effect on Carbohydrate Metabolism	Effect on Protein Metabolism	Effect on Mineral Metabolism
Estrogens	Fat deposition ketogenesis, lower cholesterolemia	Decreased	Slight anabolic	Retention of NaCl & H_2O; Ca deposition
Androgens	Little	Little	Anabolic (effect enhanced in some synthetics)	Ca deposition
Progesterone	?	?	?	Na and K retention
Adrenal mineralocorticoids				Retention of Na; loss of K
Adrenal glucocorticoids	Catabolism, liberation of NEFA	Slight anabolic Anabolic (inhibition of oxidation, enhanced gluconeogenesis)	Slight anabolic Catabolic	Slight Na retention
Insulin	Anabolic (formation of fat from carbohydrate)	Anabolic (glycogenesis) Catabolic (increased oxidation)	Anabolic (protein-sparing)	Redistribution of K, PO_4, water
Growth hormone	Catabolic	Anabolic (inhibition of oxidation, enhanced gluconeogenesis)	Catabolic in fasting. Anabolic with adequate protein, thyroxine, insulin	Slight Na, K retention
Thyroxine	Catabolic (large or continued doses)	Catabolic	Anabolic (small doses) or catabolic (large doses)	Slight Na loss; loss of Ca
Glucagon	Catabolic	Catabolic (glycogenolysis)	Slightly catabolic	?
Epinephrine	Catabolic	Catabolic (glycogenolysis)	?	?
Parathyroid	?	?	Catabolic	Ca, PO_4 withdrawal from bones; increased renal tubular Ca reabsorption and decreased PO_4 reabsorption
Thyrocalcitonin				Ca deposition in bones
ACTH	Catabolic	(Secretion of glucocorticoids)	(Secretion of glucocorticoids)	(Secretion of glucocorticoids, and some electrocorticoid effect)
Angiotensin II	?	(Secretion of electrocorticoids)	(Secretion of electrocorticoids)	(Secretion of electrocorticoids)

sive hormones are present in small quantities. Thyroid and adrenocortical hormones are prime examples.

The complexity of the interrelationships are not only a function of concentration, but often of exquisite timing. The sexual cycle of the female is the classic example. Lactation, however, probably involves greater organization. In order for lactation to occur, the lactatory ducts must be grown by estrogen, the glands grown by progesterone, milk ejection stimulated by oxytocin, and lactation induced by LTH. At the same time, fat, protein, carbohydrates, water, and so forth must be mobilized and manufactured into milk. Thyroid must be present for the cells to function properly, and the parathyroid must mobilize the large amounts of calcium needed.

From a teleological viewpoint, most of the interrelationships have a physiological explanation based on control of homeokinetic processes or mobilization of body resources for stress resistance. However, many processes do not fall into this category. In fact, some appear to represent deleterious actions on the body economy. The catabolic action of corticoids on protein in stress situations is an example, as is the antagonism of GH and insulin in carbohydrate metabolism.

From an overall viewpoint, the body can be considered as a closed system in which the output is essentially equal to the input but in which entropy increases and energy is lost as heat. The system as a whole is irreversible, but energy can be organized and stored as in adenosine triphosphate (ATP). In small subsystems, the cells are also able to increase the system's internal energy by moving materials against a gradient, by synthesizing highly organized structures such as genes, and by storing energy in fats and glycogen.

The endocrine system is the principal means of maintaining homeokinesis and keeping the increase of entropy to a minimum by its coordination of all activity.

The value of the transfer function of the contol systems as a whole must be enormous. Small sensory inputs in the order of microwatts are able to effect major changes in energy distribution *within* the organism, although the output as heat and other degraded substances is remarkably constant.

Perhaps of equal or greater importance to the organism are the control processes. The sensory system accumulates information, and functions as an input to the control systems, which are able to regulate metabolic processes to maintain homeokinesis in the face of changing environmental patterns. This overall function requires that we look at the endocrine system as a whole, rather than at each gland separately.

In the following we must examine each gland and its effect on metabolism. It must be kept in mind that every gland affects metabolism to some degree, and thus the overall effect can be explained only as the sum of these actions.

References

Bardin, C. W. and L. P. Bullock. "Testicular Feminization: Studies of the Molecular Basis of a Genetic Defect." *J. Invest. Derm.* **63** (1974): 75.

Cahn, L. and B. W. O'Malley. "Mechanism of action of the sex steroid hormones." *N. Eng. J. Med.* **294** (1976): 1322.

Cuatrecasas, P. "Insulin Receptor of Liver and Fat Cell Membranes." *Fed. Proc.* **32** (1973): 1838.

De Sombre, E. R., S. Smith, G. E. Block, D. J. Ferguson, and E. V. Jensen. *Cancer Chemother. Rep.*

Garren, L. D., G. N. Gill, H. Masui, and G. M. Walton. *Rec. Progress Horm. Res.* **27** (1971): 433.

Litwack, G. and D. Krtichevsky. *Actions of Hormones on Molecular Processes.* New York: John Wiley & Sons, 1964.

McGuire, W. L., G. C. Chamness, and R. E. Shepherd. *Life Sci.* **14** (1974): 19.

O'Malley, B. W. and A. R. Means. *Science* **183** (1974): 610.

Raspe, G. *Steroid Hormone Receptors.* Oxford: Pergamon Press, 1970.

4
The Pituitary and Hypothalamus

THE PITUITARY

The pituitary (hypophyseal)–hypothalamic system is one of the major control systems of the body. The secretions of these two so closely interrelated, yet separate organs, have major influence on the other endocrine organs, on growth and development, and on the somatic cells of the body.

In a book concerned with integration and control, the pituitary must come first in the endocrine hierarchy. A minimum amount of anatomy is essential to an understanding of physiological activity; this will be discussed next.

The pituitary (or hypophysis) has attracted attention since the time of Galen (200 A.D.). Despite its long history, it was not until 1885 that Schaefer and Oliver described some of the secretory properties of this organ. The anterior pituitary is so important, because of its influence upon many of the other endocrine organs, that it has been called the *master gland* of the body. This term is inaccurate because many endocrine organs are not under pituitary control and the others are controlled only in rate and can secrete small amounts of their characteristic products in the absence of the pituitary.

Anatomy. The pituitary in the human being is located in a cavity of the sphenoid bone, the *sella turcica*, below the base of the brain. It is attached to the brain proper by means of a stalk, the *infundibulum*. The gland is a reddish-gray mass weighing about 0.5 grams. The gland is anatomically divided into three parts; the anterior lobe or adenohypophysis, the intermediate lobe, and the posterior lobe or neurohypophysis.

The blood supply to the hypophysis is extensive and arises from the hypophysial arteries, which are branches of the carotids and the circle of Willis. These branches form an extensive capillary network upward into the hypothalamus and downward into the gland proper. Thus, the gland obtains blood directly from the arterial system and from a hypothalmico-hypophysial portal system. The dual supply has important consequences on the activity of the gland. The two major divisions, the anterior and the posterior lobes, have separate blood supplies; insofar as can be determined, they are not related functionally except in the way that all adjacent structure are interrelated. There is little indication of important innervation of the anterior pituitary, although some nerves have been demonstrated by staining. The posterior pituitary is almost entirely nervous tissue.

Histology. (See Figure 4.1.) Different cell types can be distinguished in the normal pituitary on the basis of their affinity for various dyes: acidophilic cells (alpha, including those accepting azocarmine, and orange-G dye as well as eosin); basophilic (beta) cells; and chromphobic cells. It should be emphasized that reliability of the staining and examination methods have been in considerable dispute. The fixative, the preparation of the tissue, the alkalinity of the medium, and the method of staining all appear to produce variations in the staining properties of the cells.

On the basis of changes that occur in the staining of pituitary cells of glands removed following experimental procedures, individual cell types have been assigned roles in the production or storage of specific hormones. The evidence for the type of cell responsible for production or storage of a particular hormone is based on three lines of investigation:

1. Change in normal pattern of cell types seen in an animal in which hormone production has been stimulated. For example,

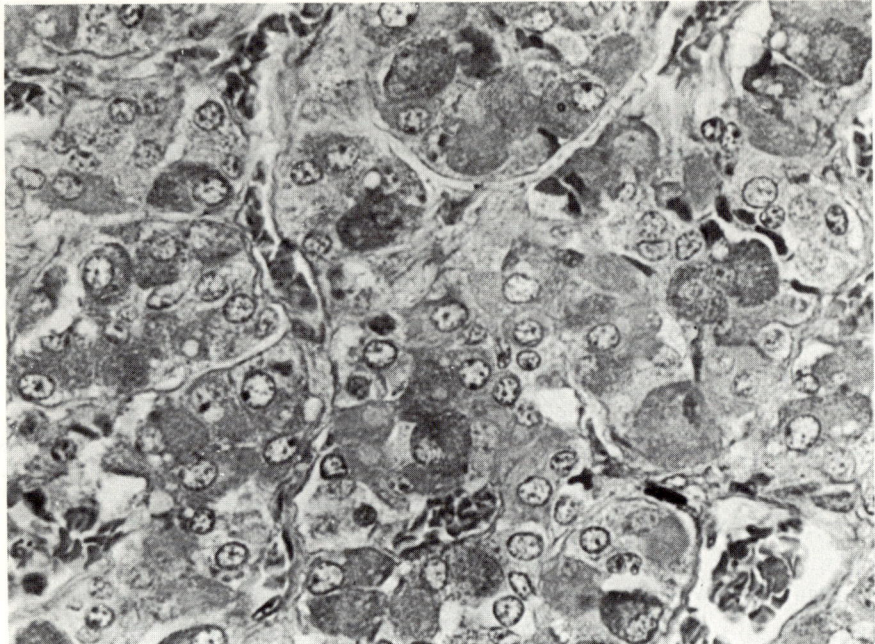

Figure 4.1. Human anterior pituitary with mallory-Azan stain after fixation in Zenker-formol; cell types are not colored differentially by a routine stain such as hematoxylineosin. The cytoplasm of acidophils (present at the upper right and lower left), which is deep red in the original slide, appears black in this photograph. Chromophobes predominate in the field and have cytoplasm lacking granules; these cells are gray in the photograph. Basophil cells are much less frequent and are larger than the chromophobes. Two basophils are seen in the same cell cord located just below the center of the photograph. Cytoplasm of the basophils is blue in the original and appears gray-black in the photograph. (Photomicrograph courtesy of Dr. R. W. Mowry.)

coitus in the rabbit causes ovulation within 1 hour; at this time there is a discharge of basophilic granules from pituitary cells, which probably contain LH. Later, luteotrophic secretion is associated with loss of carmine-staining acidophil cells.

2. The pattern of cell types can be correlated with known storage or production of specific hormones. Castration results in a large production of follicle-stimulation gonadotrophin, and it can be shown that this is related to an increased proportion of markedly degranulated and vacuolated basophils, the *signet*

ring or *castration* cells. Similar, yet not identical, changes follow thyroidectomy. ACTH overproduction can be associated with the development of a basophilic tumor of the pituitary.
3. Specific histochemical reactions can be applied to pituitary tissue. Certain of the trophic hormones are glycoprotein in nature, and a fairly specific test is available for detection of glycoprotein.

From the varied evidence, acidophilic cells contain STH (orangeophils) and luteotrophin (carminophils) and that basophilic cells contain TSH, FSH, LH, and probably ACTH. In the case of the latter two, acidophils may also be involved. There has been considerable argument as to whether all of the cell types from the pituitary are of a single origin and whether there is an interconversion of one into the other under conditions of hyper- or hypo-secretion. Chromophobes can apparently be transformed into acidophiles or basophiles, which may in turn return to the chromophobic condition, because the characteristic stainable granules are lost during the secretion process. In fact, some anatomists believe that individual cell types exist for each hormone, but this does not account for the obvious interactions that occur in the form of simultaneous secretion of hormones. Electromicroscopy has assisted in delineation of the cell types as secreting or resting cells can be identified by submicroscopic structure.

The histology of the other two lobes of the pituitary is much more clearly delineated. The posterior lobe consists of cells of nervous origin. Many nonmyelineated nerve cells, pituicytes (neuroglia), and blood vessels are arranged in a tightly packed mass.

THE HORMONES OF THE ANTERIOR PITUITARY

Removal of the anterior pituitary can be accomplished with relative ease in rats and with greater difficulty in dogs and human beings. In all species, the results are essentially the same:

1. The gonads and accessory sex organs atrophy, and their function ceases.
2. The thyroid decreases in size, and the metabolic rate decreases.
3. The adrenal gland becomes smaller due solely to atrophy of the

cortex, and the secretion of the adrenal steroids drops to low levels.
4. In the immature animal, growth ceases; there is failure to maintain body size and hair structure in the adult.
5. Disturbances occur in carbohydrate, fat, and protein metabolism.
6. There is a failure of lactation in females if hypophysectomy is performed after fertilization and before delivery.

Despite these radical changes, removal of the pituitary is not usually fatal. Since the gland controls rate processes, except for the complex integration of reproductive activity, all of the target endocrine organs continue to secrete at a low rate. This may be incompatible with life if the organism is exposed to stressful conditions, but under protected conditions, a long life is possible.

Clinically, disturbances similar to those listed above are caused by a spontaneous lack of secretion of one or more pituitary trophic hormones. Each situation can be duplicated by the failure of the trophins (with the exception of somatotrophin) to stimulate the target endocrines or by failure of the final target tissues to respond. A great deal of differential endocrinologic diagnosis is directed toward precise evaluation of these disorders.

Six adenohypophysial hormones have been isolated, five in a very highly purified form. All are known to be protein or polypeptide in nature, but with wide variation. (See Table 1.1.) Their chemistry will be discussed briefly, followed by a more detailed consideration of their individual biological actions. Some aspects of control of secretion will be discussed in the section on the hypothalamus, while still others will be discussed under sections on the target organs.

Activity of the Trophic Hormones. Growth hormone (GH) is often called somatotrophin (STH) to emphasize that it acts directly upon the peripheral tissues of the body. It is a true protein, with molecular weights varying from 21,500 in the human GH to 48,000 for ovine and bovine preparations. All have phenylalanine as both N-terminal and C-terminal amino acid, but there is a bridging in bovine and ovine materials that results in a second N-terminal sequence opening with alanine. Human GH has only two S-S bridges; most others have three or four, except for sheep GH, which has five, suggesting considerable

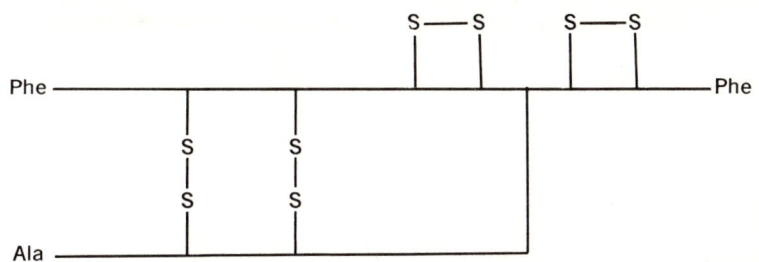

Figure 4.2. Possible structure of high molecular weight somatotrophin. As discussed in the text, the upper chain would have a molecular weight of 25,000 and is essential for activity, whereas the alanine branch would not contribute much activity.

internal bridging. Schematically, the higher molecular weight material may appear as in Figure 4.2.

The rat, mouse, and dog show a growth response to preparations from a variety of species, whereas humans respond only to primate material. A variable degree of loss of activity occurs when tryptic, peptic, or other enzymatic digestion is carefully carried out on various GH preparations, so that identification of the essential functional "core" of the molecule has not yet been possible. The results do indicate that HGH (human growth hormone) can remain active after losing 50 amino acids from the N-terminal or the C-terminal phenylanine.

P. E. Smith, H. M. Evans, and many others have demonstrated that hypophysectomized animals fail to grow. Evans performed a classic experiment in which two dachshunds were hyopophysectomized; one was treated with growth hormone and grew to be twice the size of the normal controls without losing the characteristic bodily configuration. The hormones appear to affect the growth of bone, the laying down of protein, and carbohydrate and fat metabolism. (See Table 4.1). Animals deprived of STH by hypophysectomy, and then maintained by force-feeding so that their dietary intake is equal to that of normal controls, may gain weight and size, but close examination of the process reveals that the weight deposition is largely in the form of fat, that little protein is laid down, and that the skeleton fails to mature or increase in size.

Despite the profound influence of STH on growth, some tissues appear not to be under the control of this hormone. Adrenal re-

Table 4.1. Various actions of growth hormone on tissues of the young growing rat.

Effect Measured	Control	Growth Hormone Administration
Rate of urea formation (mg N/100 gm body weight) after hydrolysate administration	8.1	5.0
Width of tibial cartilage plate (micra)	163	244
Nitrogen content (mg/gm wgt)	16.2	19.3
Weight gain (gm/day)	1.1	2.4
Rate of protein synthesis (mg N/100 gm body weight/day)	78	98
Incorporation of C^{14} into fatty acids (counts/min/mg C)	2,835	239
Rate of ketone body formation (mg % rise in blood ketones)	2.1	5.4

generation takes place in the hypophysectomized as well as the normal rat with or without GH. Most tumors appear to grow without GH, but they are also unresponsive to other hormones.

The response to GH is influenced by other hormones. Much better and longer continued growth occurs when thyroxine is given with GH, probably due to the metabolic stimulation. Hypophysectomized animals treated with GH for long periods of time may not grow due to the failure of other hormones to maintain metabolic rate, to control certain phases of protein or carbohydrate metabolism, or to stimulate other unknown factors, which may set the stage for STH action. For example, STH will not cause growth in the depancreatized animal unless insulin is supplied. Again, the explanation may be that insulin provides the energy sources for growth. As far as growth is concerned, there is also an antagonism between the glucocorticoids produced by the adrenal cortex and STH. Although testosterone also induces nitrogen retention, as does GH, the effect is largely confined to specific muscles whereas that of STH is an overall effect.

Because of its many actions of various phases of metabolism, STH has often been called the *metabolic hormone*. STH stimulates anabolism of protein (Table 4.1), with the expected results—decreased amino-acid concentration in the blood and increased serum proteins. The oxidation of fat is increased, and, as a result, STH induces increased ketone-body production. The net effect is known as *adipokinesis*. There is a pronounced effect of STH on carbohydrate metabolism. The fasting hypophysectomized animal rapidly develops hypoglycemia with a decrease in liver glycogen. This can be reversed by the administration of adrenocortical hormone, which promotes gluconeogenesis. In addition, it can be demonstrated that the hypophysectomized dog utilizes carbohydrate more rapidly than does the normal animal. The injection of STH into the hypophysectomized dog causes decreased utilization of glucose and an increased blood sugar. Continued injection of large quantities of GH results in damage to the islets of Langerhans, due to overstimulation, and a form of permanent diabetes mellitus, *pituitary diabetes.*

In 1931, Bernardo Houssay demonstrated that diabetes of pancreatic origin in animals could be ameliorated by hypophysectomy. The procedure was successful because of the opposing action of insulin and GH secretion of the blood sugar production and utilization by the body. As might be expected, adrenalectomy also ameliorated the condition of the hypophysectomized animal by enhancing gluconeogenesis and utilization of glucose by peripheral cells. However, this action is carried out along a different metabolic pathway from that affected by insulin.

The relationship of GH to the pancreas and adrenal glands is discussed in more detail in the sections of this chapter dealing with each particular gland. The general metabolic effects of growth hormone may be summarized as:

1. Growth of long bones with increase in width of the epiphyseal cartilage.
2. Involution of gastric chief cells, salivary glands, and pancreatic acini.
3. Antagonism of some of the effects of the adrenal cortex in stress.
4. Retention of nitrogen, decreased catabolism of amino acids, and increased size of the nitrogen pools. As would be expected, this leads to decreased blood urea level. A greater utilization of administered amino acids occurs.
5. Failure to mobilize tissue protein in the absence of GH, although animals without GH absorb protein nitrogen readily from the gut.
6. Disappearance of the exquisite insulin sensitivity following

hypophysectomy and development of a form of diabetes after repeated injections of STH.
7. There is a mobilization of fat from deposits to the periphery with acceleration of fatty acid catabolism, inhibition of the rate of conversion of carbohydrate to fat, inhibition of oxidation of acetate, and, as a result of changes in fat metabolism, ketogenesis. Such adipokinetic activity of STH results in an increase in nonesterified fatty acids (NEFA) in the blood.
8. GH is necessary for the adequate secretion of milk from the mammary gland, probably due to the anabolic factors necessary for the synthesis of this complex material (galactopoietic action). It should also be mentioned again that primate GH has inherent lactogenic activity, although this does not hold for lower forms.

Control of Growth Hormone. Many of the activities of GH outlined above can be summarized in a control diagram (Figure 4.3). This diagram illustrates clearly the complex interrelationships between GH secretion stimulated by various factors and the results of increased output of the cells. From another standpoint (Figure 4.4), the effects of GH may be diagramed as a mechanism for the mobilization of energy for growth and cell activity.

Figure 4.3 illustrates the major controls of GH secretion. The central nervous system (1) through a variety of mechanisms stimulates the hypothalamus (2) to release GRF (growth-hormone releasing factor), which in turn causes the secretion of GH by the pituitary (3). Through another mechanism, blood glucose, the liver (8) or the gut (9) also triggers the hypothalamus (4) to secrete GH. Obviously, the glucose in the blood is determined not only by diet or the liver but also by insulin (7) and FFA (free fatty acid) concentrations (6), all of which appear to feed back in some manner. GH obviously affects the somatic cell (5), the pancreas (7), and adipose tissue (6). Arginine can also trigger GH release (9). The different functions of the hypothalamus (2, 4) represents the action of catacholamines and somatastatin.

Figure 4.4, on the other hand, illustrates the way in which GH can mobilize energy from several sources and channel it into storage or ready energy supply.

THE PITUITARY AND HYPOTHALAMUS   51

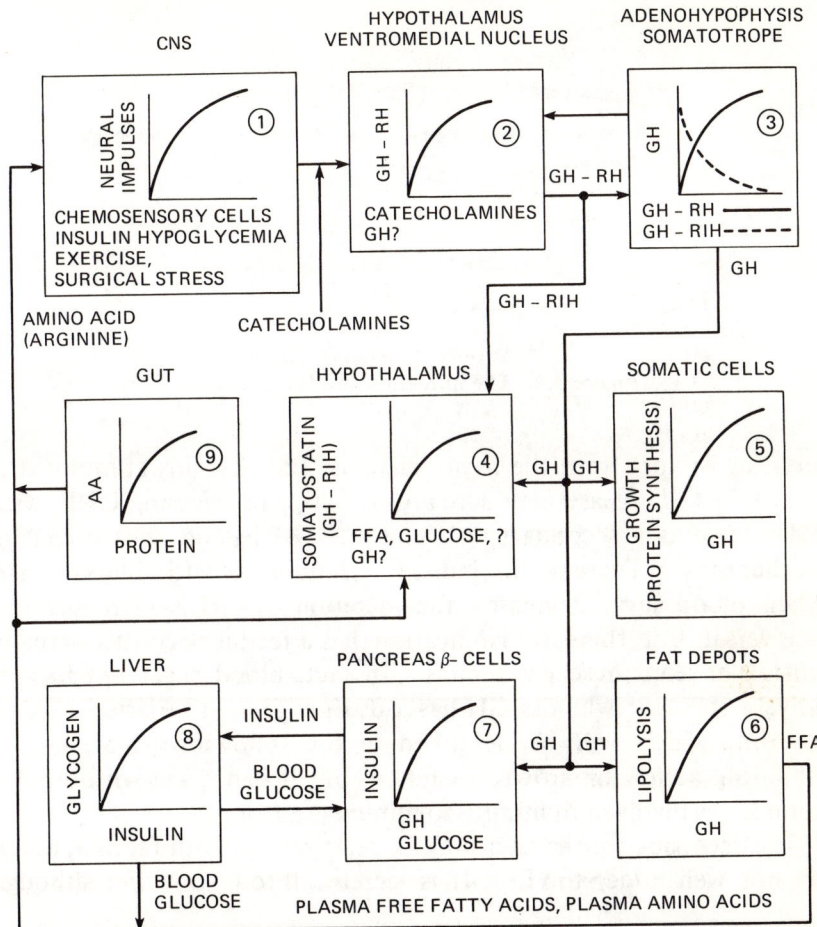

Figure 4.3. A control diagram illustrating the action of growth hormone on many locations in the body. See test for further explanation. (From J. Kline, *Biological Foundation of Biomedical Engineering*, Little, Brown, Boston, 1976, with permission.)

The release of GH is not well understood. It is clear that many factors, such as stress, starvation, and sleep, will cause its secretion (Figure 4.5, Table 4.2). Figure 4.5 is in a sense another version of Figure 4.3, illustrating the high points of the control system. It should be realized that GH release and the consequent metabolic changes are preceded by the release of GRF (growth-hormone

52 INTEGRATION AND COORDINATION OF METABOLIC PROCESSES

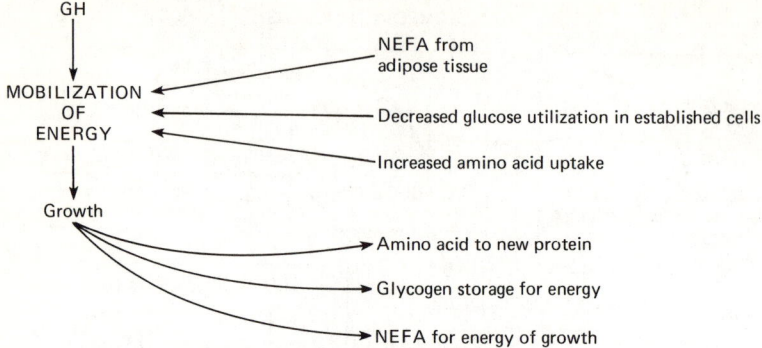

Figure 4.4. The influence of GH on growth.

releasing factor) from the hypothalamus, and that any stimulus that results in GH release may actually be active in releasing GRF, with GH release as a secondary mechanism. GH has no known control mechanisms. There is an indirect relationship with blood sugar. When blood sugar decreases, the secretion of GH is increased and vice versa. But, there is no indication that a feedback control actually exists between these parameters. In fact, blood sugar remains relatively constant whereas GH has a distinct diurnal variation. Somatostatin, which will be described in the following pages, has an inhibiting action or growth secretion, but it is not known how this hormone is involved in minute-to-minute control.

The feedback mechanism may be related to growth factors, which are not well understood. GH is secreted throughout life, although

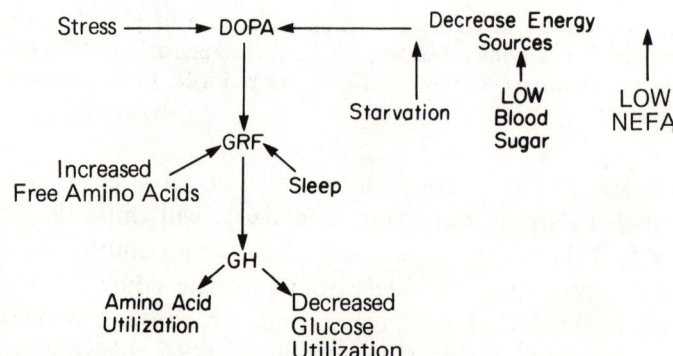

Figure 4.5. Mechanisms of release of growth hormone.

Table 4.2. Factors that stimulate GH secretion in primates.

Physiological	Biochemical	Pathological
1. Exercise	1. Insulin	1. Acromegaly
2. Stress	2. Amino-acid infusions	a. TRH
3. Sleep	3. Peptides	b. LRH
4. Decreased glucose levels	a. Vasopressin	c. Glucose
	b. -MSH	d. Arginine
	c. ACTH	2. Pyrogens
	d. Glucagon	3. Protein depletion
	4. Monadrenergic stimuli	4. Fasting and starvation
	a. Epinephrine β-receptor stimulation	
	b. L-dopa	
	c. 5-hydroxytryptophan	
	d. Melatonin	
	5. Other hormones, insulin	
	a. Estrogens	
	b. Diethylstilbestrol	
	6. Potassium infusion	

growth stops at an early age. There has been some supposition that continued secretion is necessary for cell growth and replacement. In children suffering from protein deficiency, GH secretion is increased, which may reflect the end product of feedback mechanism. GH secretion is also increased during the first 90 minutes of sleep; whether this has anything to do with cell repair is unknown.

The hypothalamus produces an oligopeptide, which specifically *inhibits* the release of GH as well as LTH and TSH. The hormone has been named *somatostatin*. It reduces GH levels markedly in acromegaly. Its main effects may well be the effects on the islet tissue of the pancreas because it also specifically inhibits *both* insulin and glucagon. In diabetes, where the insulin is already low, somatostatin reduces the level of glucagon, which in turn reduces the blood sugar.

GH stimulates the liver to produce another hormone, *somatomedin*, which has been called the *sulfation factor*. It causes an uptake of S^{32} (radioactive sulfur) in bone, which is an indication of the laying down of chrondroitin, which is part of the bone matrix. Somatomedin appears to be a protein that is similar to insulin in structure; perhaps because of the similarity, it will cause lipolysis in tissue. As would be expected, somatamedin levels are elevated in cases of acromegaly.

GH is closely related to the feeding habits of animals. Insulin is secreted in response to increased glucose blood levels, and fat and carbohydrate storage are promoted. As the level of glucose after a meal begins to fall, GH secretion is triggered; this promotes protein anabolism from the excess energy supply. Finally, GH begins to mobilize fat to NEFA, which in turn restricts the GH through unknown mechanisms. However, an interesting supposition is that low GH level does not trigger NEFA formation in the obese as readily as in the nonobese.

The basic assay of GH is relatively simple. Two methods are in general use:

1. Growth of hypophysectomized animals following injection of STH. In this assay, the growth rate in grams per day of 100 grams of body weight of hypophysectomized rats is determined over a 10-day period.
2. Increased width of the proximal epiphyseal cartilage of the tibia of hypophysectomized rats injected with GH.

Preparations of GH are usually assayed in terms of micrograms of a preparation required to produce a desired effect as compared to a standard powder arbitrarily assigned an international unit of potency per milligram. With the advent of radioimmunoassay, GH assay has become a routine matter. The young adult secretes about 385 micrograms per day. Average blood levels may reach 80 nanograms per milliliter.

Diseases of the pituitary in the human being can result either in over- or under-production of the hormone. The clinical picture is dependent upon the time at which the lesion occurs. In the child, overproduction results in gigantism without distortion of the normal growth pattern. In the adult, most of the epiphyseal junctions are closed, and overproduction of the hormone causes growth of the terminal parts of the bones, hands, feet, frontal bone, and jaw. This produces the overt signs of acromegaly (*acro*, "terminal"; *megaly*, "enlargement"). Since this is a true hyperfunction of the pituitary, many symptoms related to hyperfunction of other organs stimulated by the pituitary might be expected, and these actually occur. Many such acromegalics have enlarged thyroid glands, diabetes, and derangement of sexual function.

Conversely, hypofunction of the pituitary can also occur. In the child, the resulting decrease in metabolism and the absence of GH results in dwarfism; the person may be perfectly formed for the age at which the lesion occurred but does not grow during succeeding years. In the adult, hypofunction of the pituitary usually results in hypofunction of all of the organs regulated by the anterior lobe, "panhypopituitarism."

TSH (Thyroid-Stimulating Hormone)

Removal of the pituitary results in a decrease in metabolic rate. Injection of anterior pituitary extracts will restore the metabolic rate to normal and to greater-than-normal levels if the injections are prolonged. These effects are primarily due to pituitary thyrotrophin. As will be seen later, adrenocortical activity is also necessary in some species for full TSH action. In the normal animal, TSH is secreted at a level that maintains a normal basal metabolic rate (BMR) and cellular activity.

It can be demonstrated *in vitro* that TSH is inactivated by the thyroid gland. In normal individuals, only small amounts of the hormone can be detected in the plasma. In the hyperthyroid animal, no TSH can be found, probably due to the combination of decreased secretion by the pituitary (feedback inhibition if the hyperfunction is located at the level of the thyroid) plus increased destruction by the overactive thyroid tissue. In the absence of the thyroid, the destruction of TSH is relatively slow, and larger amounts can often be detected in the plasma. This again is due to a combination of factors—increased production from the pituitary as a result of removal of inhibition imposed by the thyroid hormone, and the absence of tissue to destroy the increased amount.

Purified TSH is readily assayed by a variety of experimental procedures, although many difficulties may attend application of the procedures to plasma, urine, or other biological material. Usually, the test involves the administration of the preparation, followed by testing of the response of the thyroid gland. There are three tests currently in use:

1. The uptake or turnover of radioiodine (I^{131}) is measured in an animal given TSH. The rate at which iodine enters the gland can also be measured. Both methods are in use and obviously determine different activities of TSH on the thyroid.

2. The epithelial cell height of the acinar cells of the thyroid can be measured following injection of TSH, preferably in repeated doses.
3. TSH-induced increase in the circulating thyroid hormone can be measured as an elevated-plasma, protein-bound iodine (PBI^{131}). It should be apparent that injection of TSH with subsequent measure of thyroid function is valuable as a diagnostic aid. Once again, the development of radioimmunoassay techniques has lead to simple assays for TSH, although it must be remembered that, in the final analysis, only a biological assay will reveal a biological function.

TSH is assayed on the basis of the U.S. Pharmacopeia (USP) unit, which is the activity of 20 milligrams of a standard powder. The original powder was a very impure protein, and better methods have produced TSH with an activity of 40 units per milligram. Present commercial preparations are not used for treatment. Replacement therapy with thyroid powder or synthetic thyroid preparations is effective and a great deal cheaper.

It is a well-known clinical observation that many patients with hyperthyroidism develop fatty deposits and edema in the orbit of the eye, with the resultant protrusion of the eyeball called *exophthalmos*. There has been considerable speculation in the literature regarding the relation of TSH to this disease. Dobyns has claimed to be able to separate from TSH another protein, which is the "exophthalmos-producing substance" (EPS) and which in itself has no effect on metabolic rate.

There is still no adequate explanation, however, of why exophthalamos may not develop until after the hyperthyroid condition has been repaired. An assumption can be made that the overactive thyroid destroys both the exophthalmic and TSH factors, and, when the gland is lowered to normal activity, there is continued production, but decreased destruction, of EPS.

ADRENOCORTICOTROPHIN (ACTH)

ACTH is a polypeptide of 39 amino acids arranged in a straight chain. Highly purified materials prepared from ovine, porcine, bovine, and human sources seem to display differences only in amino acids 25 to

33. Intensive synthetic effort has produced many peptides of the proper sequence, with the entire chain of 30 finally attained in 1963. The first 23 amino-acid units, from the N-terminal serine, was found by Hofmann to have the full activity of the entire chain. This suggests that ACTH activity in all species is produced by the identical 23-member polypeptide. Studies have indicated that ACTH protein isolated from the pituitary may be separated into two fractions α and β, with about the same molecular weight of 4,500. The latter, which is highly active, has been the material used for amino-acid composition studies. When the characteristic free groups were masked (the serine NH_2 formulation), the material was inactive as ACTH.

In the hypophysectomized animal, the function of the adrenal cortex decreases rapidly. The gland decreases in size, the atrophy being confined to the inner zones, the *zona reticularis* and *zona fasiculata*. The glomerulosa does not appear to be greatly affected by lack of ACTH. Control of overproduction of ACTH by therapy with hydrocortisone indicates the plasma level of the steroid hydrocortisone acts in a regulatory capacity to control the level of secretion of ACTH by the pituitary. ACTH is inactivated by many tissues of the body.

When the amino-acid sequence was determined for the melanocyte-stimulating hormone (MSH) from the *pars intermedia* of animal pituitaries, it was found to be the same as that of the first 13 amino acids from the N-terminal serine in ACTH. Increased pigmentation has long been recognized in Addison's disease (adrenocortical insufficiency), in which excess endogenous ACTH would be expected, and has also been noted after surgical excision of hyperfunctional adrenocortical tissue. Even though MSH has its most marked effects on the melanophores of amphibia, it is probable that this 13-amino-acid sequence influences skin pigmentation in humans.

There are several methods of assay of ACTH, all based upon the response of the target organ. Some may be considered as more direct measures of the hormone activity than others:

1. The output of steroids by the adrenals of test animals upon injection of ACTH.
2. The Sayers test, which is based upon the depletion of ascorbic acid in the adrenal cortex under ACTH stimulation, is no longer used.

3. The maintenance of adrenal weight by ACTH in the hypophysectomized rat is relatively insensitive.
4. The decrease in circulating eosinophils, which occurs following ACTH-stimulated production of adrenal steroids in most animals, has also been used but is highly nonspecific.

Once again, radioimmunoassay techniques are available for a rapid convenient assay with the aforementioned caveats.

ACTH is assayed on the basis of an international standard of ACTH (LA-1-A), which is defined as containing 1 unit per milligram. Many preparations are available that contain as high as 200 such units per milligram.

The close interrelationship among hormones is well illustrated by ACTH. The adrenal cortex of the hypophysectomized animal becomes almost unresponsive to ACTH after a short time unless thyroid hormone is given to increase the metabolic rate.

Although ACTH is by definition the hormone that stimulates the adrenal cortex, there is increasing evidence that it also plays an important extraadrenal role. It is well established that injection of ACTH into adrenalectomized animals causes a rise in plasma (NEFA). Also, ACTH increases production of NEFA from epididymal fat pads in an *in vitro* system. Although there are no other endocrines added to such an experiment, permissive amounts of corticosteroids may have been present.

Gonadotrophins. The pituitary gonadotrophins consist of three hormones that have been isolated and reasonably well purified:

FSH (follicle-stimulating hormone)
LH (luteinizing hormone; identical with ICSH, interstitial cell-stimulating hormone)
LTH (luteotrophic hormone, prolactin, lactogenic hormone, mammotrophin, and so on).

LH or ICSH is somewhat similar to FSH because it is a glycoprotein, having a molecular weight of about 25,000 and containing the same carbohydrates. However, it occurs in two chromatographically different forms (α and β), and there is little immunological cross-reaction from species to species. Human LH, recently purified, differs considerably from the others and is more active on bioassay. Some considerable argument exists as to whether FSH and LH are a single protein with activity determined by the receptors at the cellular level.

Luteotrophin (LTH) is also known as prolactin, lactogenic hormone, and mammotrophin. The purified beef and sheep preparations are proteins with molecular weights of about 25,000 and contain 205 amino acid residues, but no carbohydrate. Lysines found in the chain are essential, since acetylation blocks LTH activity. There are six linked cystines, one serving as C-terminal. All human LTH thus far isolated has exhibited lactogenic effects, although in varying quantities.

Other gonadotrophin preparations, not necessarily of pituitary origin, include human chorionic gonadotrophin (HCG), anterior pituitarylike substance (APL), and pregnant mare serum (PMS). The physiology of these hormones will be discussed under the specific target organ.

Insofar as is known, the hormones isolated from the pituitary are identical in both sexes, although there is no evidence for secretion of sex hormones other than FSH and ICSH in the male. The molecular weight varies enormously from species to species as does the chemical reactivity and antigenicity.

FSH. FSH causes growth and estrogen secretion of the ovarian follicles, but not their maturation. LH is synergistic to FSH, and this property is utilized in one assay of the hormone. The secretion of FSH by pituitary is apparently inversely related to the circulating estrogen level. In the absence of estrogen production by the ovary, the release of FSH is high, and large amounts are present in the blood and urine. This fact is taken advantage of in the assay of ovarian function in suspected ovarian failure (menopause). In the male, FSH stimulates the production of sperm if small amounts of androgen are present. It has been suggested that FSH production in the male is controlled by the small amount of estrogen secreted by the Sertoli's cells of the testes.

The hormone can be readily assayed, and two methods are in widespread use. The weight response of the ovary of a test animal to gonadotrophin is followed with or without the use of LH as a synergist. The use of LH to increase the response of the test animal to FSH was first proposed by Steelman and Pohley. The uterine weight of the immature mouse may also be used as the test object. This test response depends upon the production of estrogen by the ovary with consequent uterine response and weight gain.

LH. In the normal animal, LH causes the follicle that has been previously ripened by FSH to mature, ovulate, and develop into the corpus luteum. There is some doubt as to whether this hormone is responsible for the production of progesterone from the corpus luteum in certain species (see *LTH*). Considerable evidence suggests that LH can be released from the pituitary only in the presence of a small amount of estrogen. Once estrogen has been produced from the growing follicle with a consequent stimulation of LH release, it appears likely that the LH causes greater estrogen production from the ovary (positive feedback). When the corpus luteum begins to produce progesterone, LH production is suppressed. The feedback mechanism appears to be between progesterone and the anterior pituitary, although some estrogen is necessary for optimum response.

In the male, the same hormone (LH) is called the interstitial cell-stimulating hormone (ICSH) and serves to stimulate the production of testosterone from the interstitial cells of the testes (cells of Leydig). The androgens in turn complete the servomechanism to control LH production by the pituitary. In the male, the production of androgen appears to be a continuous process much like the production of adrenocortical steroids with a continuously operating feedback mechanism; however, it is apparent that no such direct system operates in the female.

LH appears to vary in properties from species to species. It is assayed by the characteristic response of gonadal tissue and the accessory organs. The uterine weight response of the rat has been used, but it suffers from the limitation that estrogens, FSH, and perhaps outside nervous stimuli also produce changes in uterine weight. A widely adopted method that is highly specific for LH uses the weight response of the seminal vesicles and the ventral prostate of immature male rats as the assay. These organs are subject to stimulation from the androgen, which is produced only by LH in the male rat and provides a very sensitive and specific assay. The hormone can also be assayed by radioimmunoassay techniques.

LTH. LTH has not been well studied with respect to its activity. It is known that the corpus luteum formed in the rat by the actions of

FSH and LH will not secrete progesterone until LTH is released from the pituitary. This may not be true in species other than the rat; in particular, there is doubt that this is true for humans. As a lactogenic hormone, LTH is very effective in causing milk secretion from the mammary gland that has been suitably prepared with estrogen and progesterone. Its action in the male is undetermined. One of the major difficulties in studying the physiology of LTH is the lack of a convenient assay. At present, the hormone is assayed by the growth of the crop sac of the pigeon, which is its accessory sex organ.

Chorionic Gonadotrophins. Many substances have been referred to as "chorionic gonadotrophin." The name is a misnomer because some hormones of this class can be produced by the testes, but none are produced by the chorion. These gonadotrophins actually originate from the placenta in the female. Their names are not always descriptive of the site of origin: pregnant mare serum (PMS) is obtained from the plasma of the pregnant mare; anterior pituitarylike substance (APL) is obtained from the blood or urine of various primate species; and human chorionic gonadotrophin (HCG) is obtained from the urine of pregnant women. Despite some similarities of action, the hormones differ widely from each other. HCG appears to contain mostly LH-like materials. PMS, which contains both FSH-and LH-like materials, has been used to cause ovulation in women. It may not be a true gonadotrophin since it arises from the endometrium of the pregnant horse. Hormones may be obtained from testicular tumors that are either LH- or FSH-like. It should be emphasized that although these hormones behave in many respects like those derived from the pituitary, they are not identical. The chorionic gonadotrophins are found in the urine with the single exception of PMS, which apparently does not pass the kidney of the mare. Most of them contain the sugar mannose or galactose in combination with the protein moiety of the molecule. The substances disappear readily from the blood, and many of them appear to be inactivated by the liver. PMS is destroyed more slowly than are any of the others.

The many assays devised to detect chorionic gonadotrophins are the basis for all pregnancy tests since the increase in hormone production depends upon placental formation and viability. Since levels of gonadotrophin in the pregnant women can reach 100,000 units (1 unit is equal to a 100 percent increase in the weight of the uterus of a rat) per day during the first trimester, the material is relatively easy to detect. Levels decline rapidly after this time, and then the tests are not so valuable. The presence of testicular tumors of the gonadotrophin-secreting type is also recognized by the same test.

The gonadotrophins are usually assayed on the basis of a unit equal to a dose required to produce a 100 percent increase in the size of the test organ. Armour Laboratories has made available standard preparations of gonadotrophins from several species that contain about 1 unit per milligram, but there is presently no international standard. Reichert and Parlow have reported separation of relatively pure FSH containing about 25 units per milligram. Once again, radio-immunoassay techniques have simplified protein hormone assay, and, as we will see, the mass spectrometer has greatly aided those assays depending on steroid assays.

THE HYPOTHALAMUS

Secretion of Anterior Pituitary Hormones. It has been repeatedly stressed that the relationship between the level of secretion of the trophic hormone and that of the target organ is such as to maintain an adjusted function of the target organ through a feedback mechanism. However, this is not the only method of control of pituitary secretion. There are other factors, most of which are not well understood. The mating of birds under the influence of light intensity and the ovulation of the rabbit during or following coitus are specific examples. In recent years, considerable evidence has accumulated to indicate that the brain is involved in most of the "feedback" circuits between the pituitary and the target organ.

The neural secretions can be divided into two classes: the neurohumors, which are the nervous-system transmitters, acetylcholine and norepinephrine; and the neurosecretory substances, which include oxytocin, vasopressin, and other substances. The two systems together could be classed as the *neurohormones*.

Portal System of the Pituitary. This system provides an ideal location for an exchange of a neurohumoral agent between the hypothalamus and the anterior pituitary. A plexus is formed from

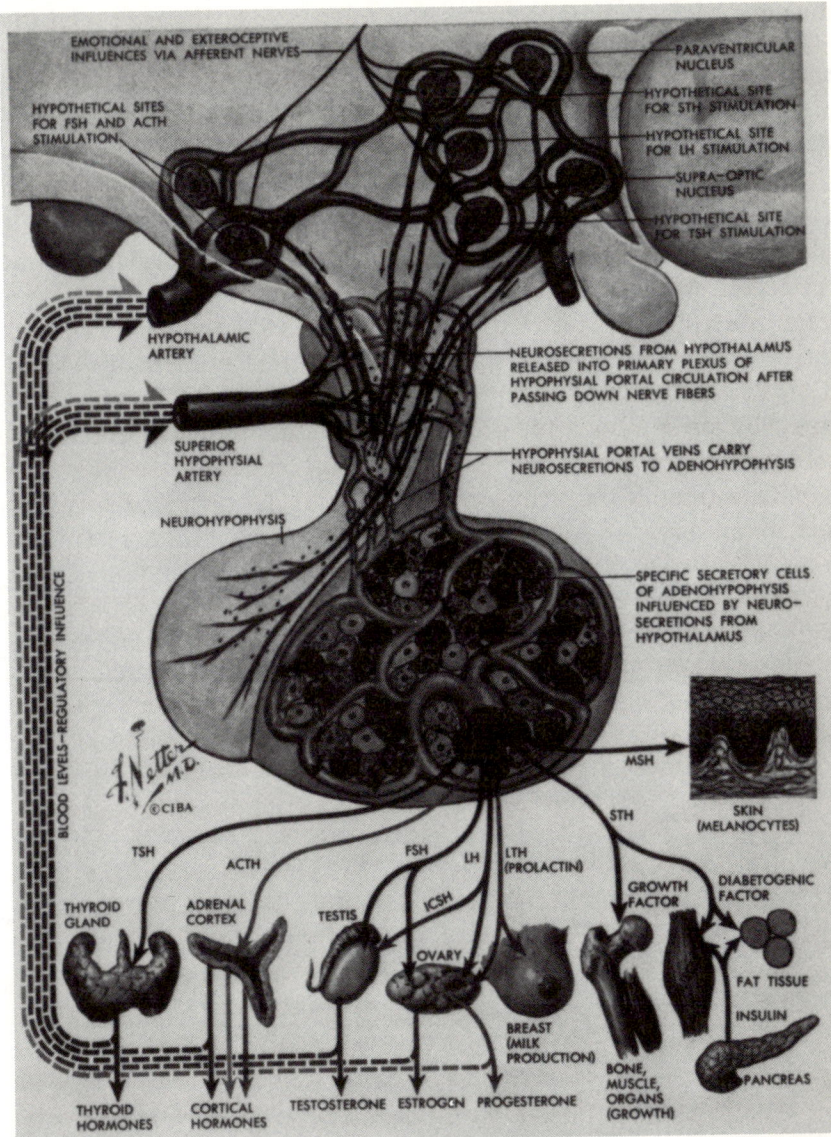

Figure 4.6. A sketch of the hypothalamus indicating the systems coordinated by this region and its circulatory connections with the pituitary. (Copyright, *The CIBA Collections of Medical Illustrations* by Frank H. Netter, M.D.)

branches of the internal carotid; this lies between the pars tuberalis and the median eminence (see Figure 4.6). Capillary loops arise from the plexus and enter the infundibulum where they are surrounded by nerve fibers from the hypothalamus. The loops then return to the plexus and drain into the sinuses of the anterior lobe.

That this system is actually physiological in nature has been well established by Geoffrey Harris. If the stalk of the pituitary is severed following coitus in the rabbit, LH is not released and ovulation does not occur. When the pituitary is severed from the remainder of the brain, even though it is left in the sella turcica, epinephrine fails to initiate the characteristic response of ACTH release. Lesions placed in the hypothalamus also appear to be able to block ACTH release initiated by stress even in the presence of an intact pituitary gland.

In summary, there is clear evidence that secretion of the individual trophic hormones from the anterior pituitary is controlled to a variable extent by the hypothalamus and that each hormone is elaborated following stimulation of a specific area of the hypothalamus (Figure 4.7). Since the hypothalamus controls a variety of functions, including cardiovascular activity, temperature regulation, hunger and thirst, gastrointestinal tone, respiration, sleep, and possibly many others, a lesion in this region is likely to produce many effects.

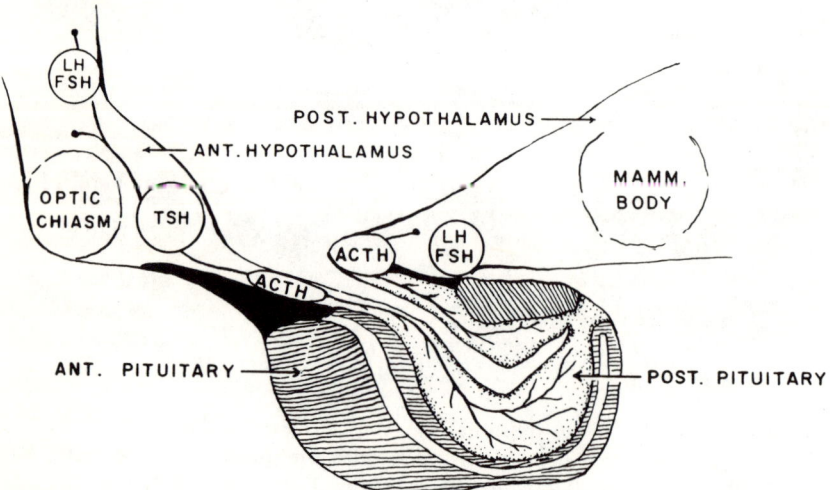

Figure 4.7. The approximate areas of the hypothalamus where electrical stimulation causes secretion of characteristic hormones from the anterior pituitary or where lesions block specific secretions.

Hypothalamic Mechanism and Mediator. The question still arises as to the mechanisms by which the hypothalamus is triggered to secrete a characteristic substance which in turn stimulates the pituitary release of each specific trophic material. Production of corticotrophin-releasing factor (CRF), for example, is apparently conditioned by many factors, but the level of circulating steroid is probably of minor importance. Release of TSH is influenced by certain nervous factors and is apparently inhibited by thyroxine.

Nervous control of gonadotrophin release was established when it was shown that rat pituitaries are spontaneously stimulated between 2 and 4 p.m. on the day preceding ovulation and that the release of gonadotrophic hormone requires about 0.5 hour. It was also shown that the process could be blocked by the use of adrenergic blocking agents. Another line of evidence was established by Critchlow when he induced ovulation of rats by electrically stimulating the hypothalamus for 30-minute periods. Furthermore, when pituitaries of normal rats were transplanted to the temporal lobes or to the median eminence of the brain, only those in the eminence elaborated gonadotrophin and permitted the continuation of normal cycles. These lines of evidence strongly suggest that the brain is responsible for triggering the secretion of gonadotrophins from the anterior pituitary, that the region responsible is sharply localized, and that no direct nervous connection is necessary for the process to occur.

The only possible explanation is the elaboration of a neurohormone from the hypothalamus, which reaches the pituitary and stimulates production of the trophic hormones. Furthermore, since ovulation occurs in a regularly timed sequence conditioned by the presence of estrogen from the ovary, the hypothalamic centers must be responsive to the level of circulating steroids produced by the ovary. Ovulation in the rabbit only occurs following the nervous stimulation of coitus, thus suggesting that nervous factors also enter into the total integrative picture. The control of LH-secretion by a hypothalamic mechanism has been demonstrated by McGann who found that LH release was *decreased* by hypothalamic lesions. However, in the rat with a pituitary transplanted to the kidney, secretion of prolactin increased even though FSH and LH secretions disappeared, indicating previous hypothalamic *inhibition* of prolactin liberation. It is apparent that both releasing and inhibiting substances are present as transmitters.

66 INTEGRATION AND COORDINATION OF METABOLIC PROCESSES

Table 4.3. The neurohormonal glands.

Gland	Secretion
Adrenal medulla	Epinephrine
	Norepinephrine
Neurohypophysis	Vasopressin
	Oxytocin
Median eminence of hypothalamus	Hypophysiotropic hormones
	Corticotropin-releasing factor (CRF)
	Thyrotropin-releasing factor (TRF)
	Somatotropin-releasing factor (SRF)
	Follicle-stimulating hormone-releasing factor (FRF)
	Luteinizing hormone-releasing factor (LRF)
	Prolactin-inhibiting factor (PIF)
	Melanocyte-stimulating hormone-inhibiting factor (MSH-IF)
Pineal gland	Melatonin
Subcommissural organ	Reissner's fiber

The neurohormones of the hypothalamus are polypeptides ranging in size from 3 to 20 amino acids (Table 4.3, Figure 4.8). Each polypeptide with minor exceptions releases or inhibits a particular pituitary hormone and operates in a typical feedback circuit (Figure 4.9).

The feedback circuits are not well understood, as illustrated by the question marks in Figure 4.9. It is clear that the target-organ hormone can suppress secretion of the proper trophin, but it is not clear whether this system operates in the brain or in the pituitary. Neither is it completely clear whether the pituitary hormone itself acts as the feedback to the hypothalamus.

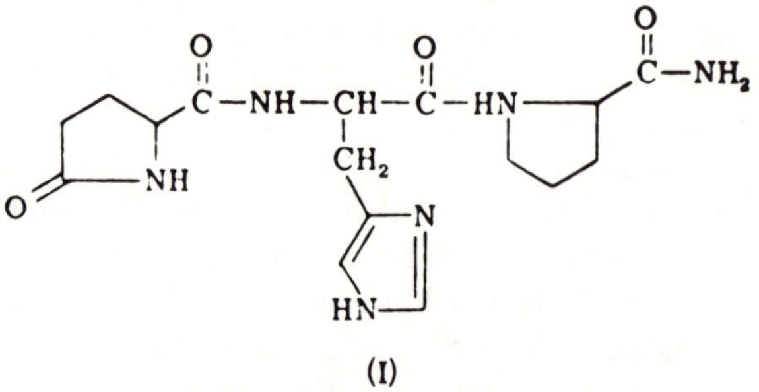

(I)

Figure 4.8. Structure of TRH.

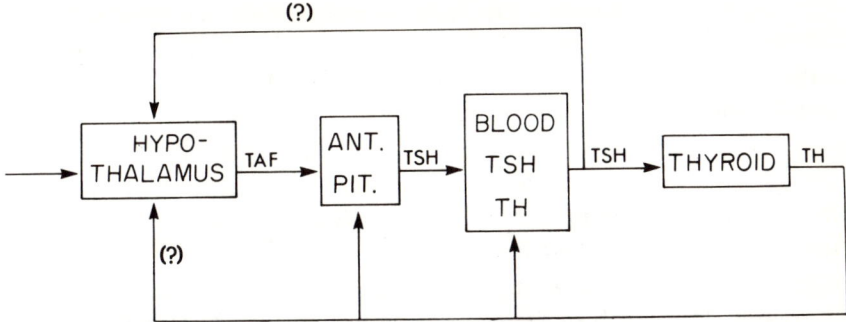

Figure 4.9. The feedback of TSH and thyroid hormone to the pituitary and hypothalamus illustrating the unknown though suspected circuits.

CRF. Many workers have shown that lesions placed in the central hypothalamus block the usual secretion of adrenocortical steroids following stress, indicating that the pituitary is no longer capable of secreting ACTH when the hypothalamus is inactive. The situation is not completely clear-cut since dogs with lesions that block output of steroids under stress do not show any signs of adrenal atrophy, which should certainly occur if ACTH were absent from the blood. This result is in marked contrast to dogs in which the connection between the hypothalamus and the pituitary is served, but in which the hypothalamus is still intact. In these animals, the adrenal undergoes marked atrophy, while the stress response remains intact.

Polypeptides have the ability to cause secretion of the adrenal cortex hormones in the presence but not in the absence of the pituitary. This material, corticotrophin-releasing factor (CRF) has been isolated. Furthermore, it can be shown that CRF in turn must be triggered by some nervous stimulus, which can be blocked by morphine. CRF is therefore assayed in the morphine-blocked intact rat. It could also be assayed in the rat in which the hypothalamic centers had been previously destroyed. It has been suggested that the feedback mechanism operates so that steroid levels control the rate of ACTH synthesis whereas the hypothalamus controls the rate of ACTH release.

TRF. The rat exposed to cold shows a much greater rate of release of I^{131} from the thyroid than does the rat not exposed, indicating that nervous stimulation has in some way triggered the output to TSH from the pituitary and stimulated greater thyroid activity. It has also been found that any type of stressful stimuli imposed upon the organism will increase ACTH output and markedly decrease TSH output. These results indicate a nervous involvement in TSH production by the pituitary. The evidence is supported by the work of Roy O. Greep, who found that lesions in the supraoptic region prevented the increase in thyroid size which usually accompanies the feeding of thiouracil. Later work established that, when the growth response of the thyroid was blocked by hypothalamic lesions, no effect could be noted on the iodide-trapping mechanism. D'Angelo has demonstrated decreased TSH levels in the blood of hypothalamic-lesioned animals.

Although nervous stimulation of the anterior pituitary may be of great physiological importance, it is not the only trigger to TSH elaboration. Thyroxin is capable of decreasing the TSH production of anterior pituitary cells transplanted to the anterior chamber of the eye. Radioactive thyroxine is rapidly accumulated by the pituitary, suggesting a direct action of the hormone on the pituitary.

Recent immunochemical studies show a rapid inverse relationship between the blood levels of glucose and TSH, but any feedback relationship is difficult to demonstrate. In fact, the elaboration of the functions of the various neurohumors have been made possible only by radioimmunoassay techniques.

Some discussion still exists as to whether LH and FSH have the same releasing factor, and some aspects of the release of these hormones suggest a common triggering mechanism.

References

Franchimont, P. and H. Burger. *Human GH and Gonadotrophins in Health and Disease.* Amsterdam: North Holland Publishing, 1975.

Goth, E. and J. Favengi. *Polypeptide Hormones.* Budapest: Hungarian Academy of Sciences, 1971.

Gray, C. H. and A. L. Bacharach. *Hormones in Blood.* 2 vols. New York: Academic Press, 1967.

Gual, C. and E. Rosenburg. *Hypothalamic–Hypophysiotrophic Hormones.* Amsterdam: Excerpta Medica, 1973.

Litwak, G. *Biochemical Actions of Hormones.* No. 1, 1970; No. 2, 1972; No. 3, 1975. New York: Academic Press, 1975.

Locke, W. and A. V. Schally. *The Hypothalamus and the Pituitary in Health and Disease.* Springfield, Illinois: Charles C Thomas, 1972.

Martini, L. and W. F. Ganong. *Frontiers in Neuroendocrinology.* New York: Raven Press, 1976.

McGann, S. B. *Endocrine Physiology*. Baltimore: University Press, 1975.
Pastells, J. L. and C. Robyn. *Human Prolactin*. Amsterdam: Excerpta Medica, 1973.
Quay, W. B. *Pineal Chemistry*. Springfield, Illinois: Charles C Thomas, 1974.
Szentagothai, J., B. Flerko, B. Mess, and B. Halasz. *Hypothalamic Control of the Anterior Pituitary*. Budapest: Hungarian Academy of Sciences, 1968.

5
Neurohypophysis and Other Hormonal Agents

Considerable evidence has accumulated to indicate that extracts from the posterior pituitary possess three major activities: an antidiuretic, an oxytocic, and a pressor activity. Until recently, there has been a controversy over whether one, two, or three separate hormones were produced. All of the activity of posterior pituitary extracts can be described in terms of two pure octapeptides, synthesized by Vincent Vigeneaud from component amino acids. Present evidence suggests the presence of only two hormones differing from each other by two amino-acid residues. These hormones are vasopressin, which also has the antidiuretic function, and oxytocin, which contains the oxytocic activity and is also capable of causing milk ejection in the prepared animal (Table 5.1).

Even though considerable storage of the hormones occurs in the posterior pituitary, evidence now indicates that this is not the site of production of the hormones. Ranson and others advocated for more than 20 years that the supraopticohypophysial tract regulated the secretion of the posterior pituitary because interruption of these tracts resulted in decreased production of the hormones. It was demonstrated in 1954 that isolated pituicytes produced no hormone

Table 5.1. Activity of posterior pituitary hormones on several physiological functions (expressed as units/mg).

Hormone	Vasopressor Activity	Antidiuretic Activity	Milk Ejection	Rat Uterus Contraction
Arginine Vasopressin	300	300	51	9
Lysine Vasopressin	200	24	34	5
Oxytocin	7	3	360	420

when a pituitary freshly depleted of hormone was removed from an animal for use in a tissue-culture procedure.

HORMONE PRODUCTION

From this and other evidence, it is now clear that the hormones are produced by the nerve cells of the supraoptic and paraventricular nuclei. Colloid droplets considered to be neurosecretory material flow down the axons to the posterior pituitary. If the axons are cut, stained neurosecretory material accumulates on the proximal side of the cut. It is probable that the hormonal substances pass into the posterior pituitary gland proper and are stored there until released by physiological stimuli (Figure 5.1). The hormones appear to be transported into the axon stream of the nerve cells at a slow rate since, if the gland is depleted in hormones, some time is required to replace the lost material. The mechanism as previously described has been further substantiated by the isolation from the supraoptic and paraventricular nuclei of material with high oxytocic, antidiuretic, and pressor activity.

In the posterior pituitary, the material appears to be stored in granules; when procedures are applied that decrease the stores of neurohumoral material (such as dehydration, which increases ADH secretion), empty sacs appear where densely stainable granules once existed. Release of the hormone is not easily explained. Some mechanism must cause the material to traverse the granule wall and the cell wall before it can reach the pituitary interstitial spaces. It has been proposed that the material produced in the nerve cells is a protein, neurophysine, to which the active octapeptides are

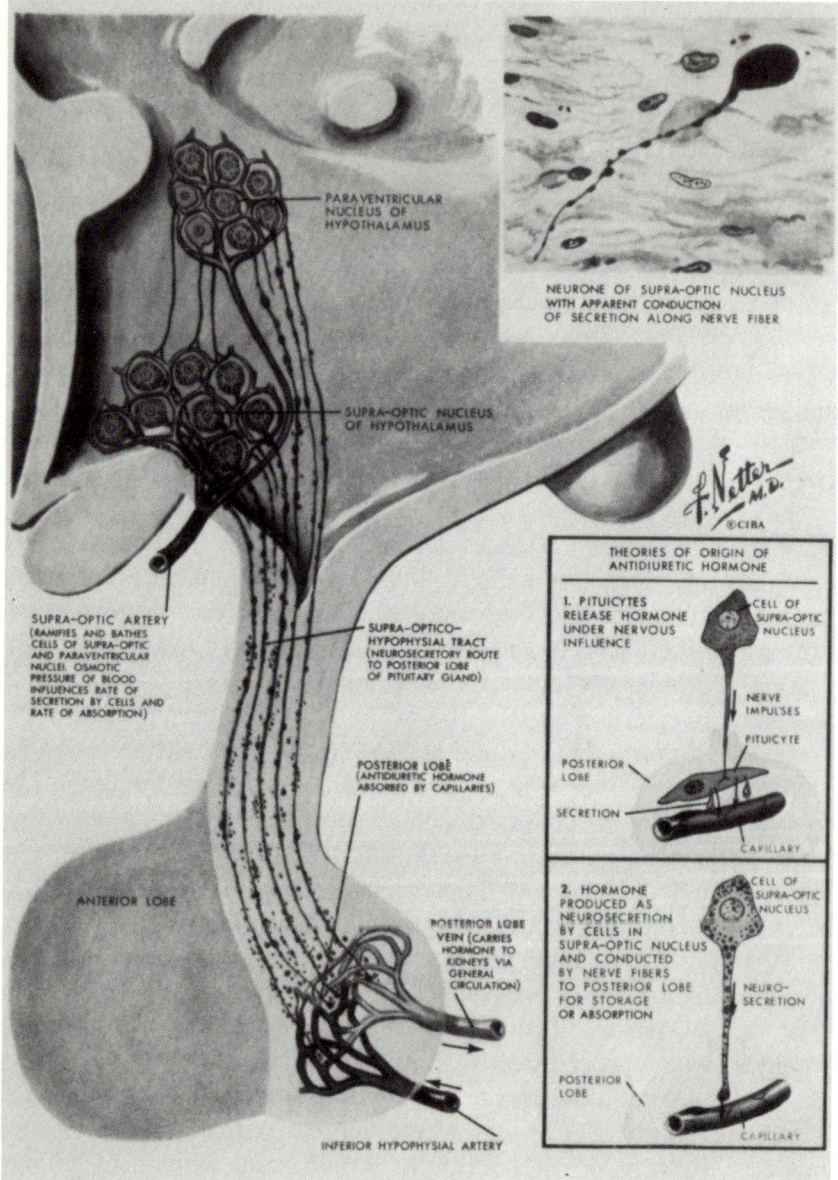

Figure 5.1. The hypothalamus and posterior pituitary, indicating the nervous and circulatory connections. (Copyright, *The CIBA Collection of Medical Illustrations* by Frank H. Netter, M.D.)

attached in equimolar proportions. If this is also the storage form of the hormones, the desired peptide might be released by a specific proteolytic enzyme.

This poses some difficulty in itself, since the isolated octapeptides are quite different in their levels of physiological activity (see Table 5.1), and it is apparent that different physiological stimuli cause the release of one or the other peptides specifically. This differing secretion ratio of oxytocin to vasopressin might be explained on the basis of storage of the hormones in their peptide form. F. S. La Bella has been able to separate granules from the posterior pituitary, each containing only one hormone. This possibility of release of one type of granule at a time offers a better explanation of the activity. Any study of secretory activity is complicated by the very rapid disappearance of the hormones from the blood when they are injected, which is not surprising, considering that they are small peptides and are undoubtedly subjected to enzymatic breakdown in the liver, the kidney, and possibly the bloodstream itself.

The Oxytocic Hormone. The influence of oxytocin on the uterus is twofold: (1) it propels sperm into and through the uterus, and (2) it propels the fetus from the uterus. Both of these activities are the result of motility of the uterus; it has been claimed that in cows the act of mating or perhaps the presence of sperm in the vagina results in the release of oxytocin and a contraction of the uterus. There is a well-known increase in motility of the pregnant uterus at term, and this can be duplicated by the injection of oxytocin. An enzyme in the blood destroys oxytocin in the normal female, but this enzyme declines in amount during the last few weeks of pregnancy, allowing greater motility of the uterus and perhaps initiating parturition.

At any rate, the uterus is exquisitely sensitive to oxytocin, with about 5×10^{-5} milligrams producing an easily detectable response (contraction). The sensitivity increases slowly during pregnancy and reaches a maximum shortly before parturition. The cervix becomes less sensitive to oxytocin during pregnancy.

In addition to its action on the uterus, oxytocin exerts a profound effect on the mammary gland. It has long been known that the destruction of portions of the hypothalamus in several species resulted in a markedly decreased milk supply to the suckling young. Lactation was restored to normal by the injection of oxytocin. This

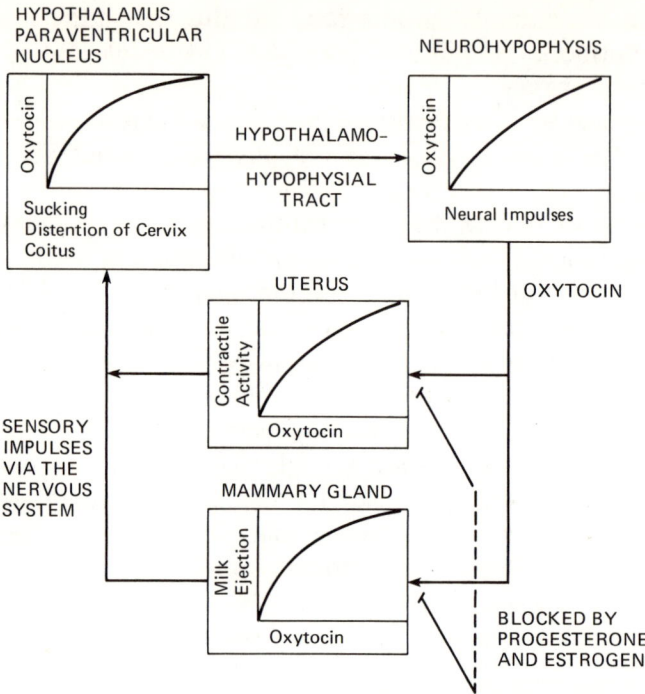

Figure 5.2. The control system for oxytocin and its action on the uterus and mammary gland. (From J. Kline, *Biological Foundation of Biomedical Engineering*, Little, Brown, Boston, 1976, with permission.)

has been named the *milk ejection effect*. Inhibition of hormone secretion is suggested in the woman where anxiety, worry, and the like has decreased the milk flow. Although the role of oxytocin in actual ejection of milk from the engorged human mammary gland is not established, it is well documented in lower animals. The control of oxytocin secretion is diagramed in Figure 5.2.

Vasopressin-Antidiuretic Hormone. The action of vasopressin as a vasopressor agent under normal conditions is not well demonstrated. Removal of the posterior pituitary does not result in any drop in blood pressure, and injection of vasopressin has only a minor effect compared to other accepted pressor materials. The action of the pressor substance appears to be largely on the smooth muscle of the circulatory system to produce a generalized vasoconstriction that is not mediated by autonomic agents or blocked by nerve section, adrenalectomy, or the usual autonomic blocking agents.

The effect is not marked in human beings and the only response to injection of the material is pallor and decreased heart rate. Large doses produce greater rises in blood pressure, but the preparation exhibits tachyphylaxis (that is subsequent doses produce smaller and smaller relative responses). Vasopressin probably has no physiological or clinical importance as a pressor agent.

The antidiuretic activity of vasopressin is of great importance. Administration of posterior pituitary extracts to animals or humans results in the retention of water and of salt; hence the term *antidiuretic hormone* (ADH). Verney has demonstrated that the major stimulus to ADH production in the normal animal is raised osmotic pressure of the intracellular fluid since injection of hypertonic solutions into the hypothalamus results almost immediately in retention of water. The *osmoreceptors* apparently do not adapt to the stimulus, since increasing the hypertonicity or the length of exposure increases the antidiuretic effect. Even when plasma sodium is below normal, ADH is capable of diminishing urine volume (Figure 5.3.).

The response may not be the simple relationship that it appears to be. Several workers have attempted to demonstrate that the controlling factor may be extracellular fluid volume rather than osmotic balance. Sudden decrease in blood volume produces a profound antidiuresis, which previously led to the theory that ADH secretion can be caused by stimulation of the baroreceptors (pressoreceptors) in the carotid sinus. The discovery of a baroreceptor control of secretion of the powerful sodium-retaining electrocorticoid, aldosterone, has introduced a complicating feature. These two factors have been combined in Figure 5.4.

The rate of ADH secretion varies considerably among species and appears to be greater in animals that must conserve water in order to live. The kangaroo rat, which lives in the desert and excretes a urine about five times as concentrated as that of the dog, has an ADH urinary excretion of 50 milliunits per day, compared to 6 milliunits per day in the dog. The posterior pituitary gland of the kangaroo rat also contains large amounts of ADH, which is reflected in the remarkable ability of this species to conserve water. The posterior pituitary of the newborn infant is extremely low in ADH, which may explain the large urinary volume and easily disturbed water balance of the child.

The action of ADH is a rapid one. The time from drinking a hypertonic saline solution to the maximum inhibition of urine flow

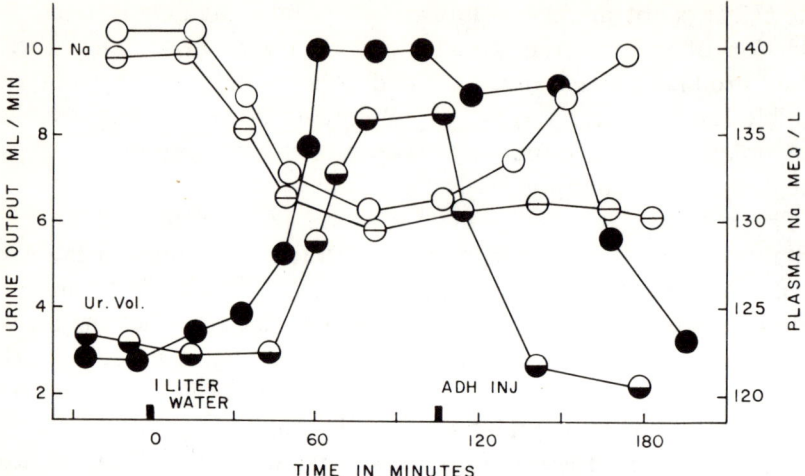

Figure 5.3. The effect of antidiuretic hormone (ADH, vasopressin) on the urine output of subjects drinking 1 liter of water in relation to the plasma concentration of sodium. The solid circles represent the urine volume of a student drinking pure water; open circles represent the data collected on his plasma sodium levels. The half-solid circles are urine-volume data obtained from another student given an injection of 0.2 milliliters of an ADH preparation at the height of diuresis, approximately 105 minutes after ingesting 1 liter of water. The barred circles represent the plasma sodium levels of the latter student given ADH. Notice that, in this case, the urine volume decreased independently of plasma sodium owing to the exogenous hormone.

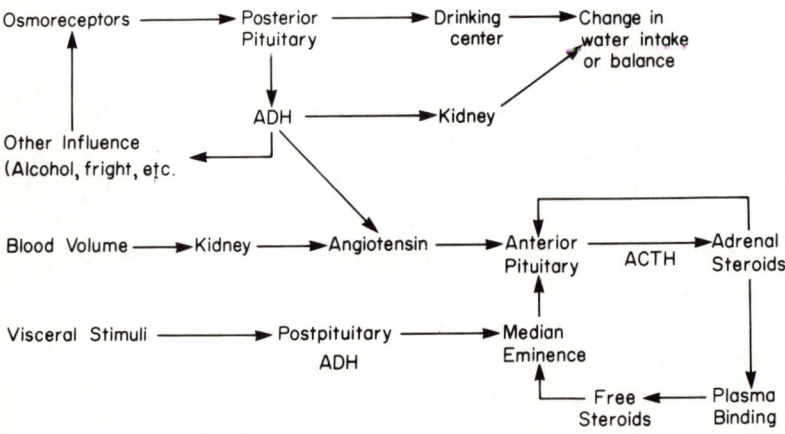

Figure 5.4. A general diagram of the ADH control system.

may be less than 0.5 hour, including absorption from the gut, secretion of ADH by the pituitary, and increased water reabsorption by the kidney. In the opposite direction, it has been estimated that a decrease of ADH concentration of one part of 10^{10} in the plasma of a human will produce diuresis.

The control of ADH secretion is complicated. Figure 5.5 illustrates the controls and their interrelationships between the kidney, adrenal, and posterior pituitary. The simpler effect of water volume or osmolarity on feedback control of ADH is shown in Figure 5.4.

The principal sites of action of ADH promoting water reabsorption are the distal convoluted tubule and the collecting duct of the nephron. This function depends upon the osmotic gradient established by the countercurrent mechanism in the loops of Henle originally demonstrated by Wirz. The importance of the thin segment is particularly well demonstrated in the kangaroo rat, which has tremendous power to concentrate urine and in which the loop of Henle is extremely long, projecting into the ureter.

Failure of the posterior pituitary system in a human produces no evidence of hormonal impairment except that attributable to ADH. The facultative reabsorption of water by the kidney is impaired, and the excretion of water may reach 20 liters per day of very dilute urine. This condition, diabetes insipidus, may persist for years with no damage if free ingestion of water is allowed. This

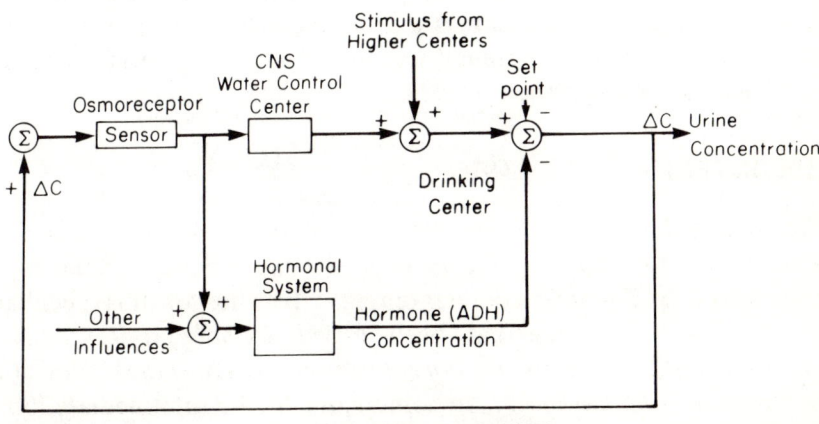

Figure 5.5. The overall control of water balance from both ADH and the adrenal.

should not be confused with diabetes mellitus, which may also involve excretion of large volumes of urine, due in this latter case to urinary loss of glucose and impaired osmotic relationships. The former disease can be completely controlled by the administration of extracts of posterior pituitary by nasal insufflation of dry powder, by injection of material in oil suspension, or by water extracts that are fully injectable. Since the active substances are polypeptidic, oral administration is not feasible. Lately, chlorpropamide and the thiazides have been found to reduce polyuria through unknown mechanisms.

Assay of the synthetic posterior pituitary hormone has taken many forms. The vasopressor fraction can be assayed by following a rise in blood pressure after intravenous injection of test material. The oxytocic principle is usually assayed by the response of the rat or guinea pig uterus to the peptide *in vitro*, although some laboratories use the depression of blood pressure in the bird following injections of the desired material. ADH is estimated by the antidiuretic response of pituitary stalk-sectioned dogs or water-loaded animals (usually rats). All of these assays suffer from difficulties that cannot be avoided. The route of injection, presence of augmentor or inhibitor material, influence of small amounts of one neurohormonal substance upon another, and other unknown factors affect the sensitivity and accuracy of the assay. Since unitage of the material is described in terms of an impure preparation of posterior pituitary gland (1 IU equals 0.5 milligrams), many preparations are available with high potency and many assays are performed in terms of microunits of the standard.

THE INTERMEDIATE LOBE

The intermediate lobe of the pituitary of many species secretes a hormone that is capable of dispersing the melanocytes of the skin to produce a characteristic darkening. Because of this peculiar property, the hormone has been called *melanocyte-stimulating hormone* (MSH), *chromatophore hormone* (CH), *intermedin*, or *intermediate-lobe hormone*. In some animals, the intermediate lobe can be easily dissected free from the other lobes and, as is the case in the mouse lobe, grown in tissue culture where it has been demonstrated that these cells produce the characteristic hormone, MSH. In most animals, the intermediate lobe is almost indistinguishable from the anterior lobe and is usually separated with it on dissection. Thus, its function cannot truly be evaluated in the classical manner.

Aside from the melanophore-expanding activity of the hormone in lower animals, especially amphibia, some metabolic effects have been reported in mammals. Although these effects should be viewed with caution until pure preparations are available and until better assays are perfected, it has been claimed that extracts of the intermediate lobe increase the metabolic exchange of mammary tissue *in vitro* from either accelerated lipogenesis or glycolysis. The extracts have also been claimed to accelerate mitosis. This has been attributed to facilitation of the glucokinase reaction and may be an indication of the activity of the hormone in some phase of glucose metabolism.

The material is a relatively low-weight polypeptide, containing 18 amino acids in linear array, which has been prepared in pure form from ox and pig posterior lobes. It was originally claimed to be identical with the "ascorbic-acid–depleting factor" of ACTH and is thought to account for the pigmentation that sometimes results from ACTH administration. Patients having adrenocortical failure (Addison's disease), with resultant high ACTH production, usually display increased pigmentation. Furthermore, melanin production is inhibited by hormones of the adrenal cortex, notably cortisol. There is also an increased pigmentation during pregnancy, which has been attributed to MSH release. By the most reliable assays, patients with Addison's disease and pregnant women excrete about 400 units per day compared with the normal excretion of 40 units per day.

There are two kinds of MSH, *alpha* and *beta*. The relationship betweeen alpha MSH and ACTH is evident from their structures, since the first 13 amino acids are identical in the two polypeptides. Lerner evaluates ACTH as having about one-thirtieth of the darkening ability of MSH and finds that the acetylation of the terminal serine-NH_2 increases this to one-fifth. The beta-sequence is not so closely related to ACTH nor does it exhibit as much activity as MSH. It is not surprising that ACTH should have MSH activity. Despite the close structural relationship, MSH has little of the adipokinetic activity of ACTH.

MSH is assayed by the response of the hypophysectomized frog to the injections of the hormone. In this test animal, the pigment-containing cells are contracted and the animal is light in color. Upon injection of an extract of intermediate-lobe material, there is immediate expansion of the melanophores, resulting in darkening of the skin, which can best be quantitated by reflectance photometry. An *in vitro* assay is also available in which excised frog skin is exposed to varying concentrations of MSH in the incubation fluid. Neither type of assay is fully satisfactory for measurement of the hormone in blood or urine because many complications, such as the inhibitory action of norepinephrine and epinephrine, have not been taken into account. Although assays have been proposed for use in pregnancy and certain other conditions, no direct action of the hormone and no clinical illness from its presence or absence are known in the human being.

MSH can be used in darkening the skin artificially. The use of salicylates in suntan lotion may act to promote rapid darkening through the release of MSH.

THE PINEAL LOBE

As more sophisticated techniques of chemical analysis have been developed in the past few years, attention has been attracted to the pineal gland as another endocrine organ. The pineal, located in the brain itself, arises from the roof of the third ventricle and is connected by a stalk of the commissures. There are few nerve fibers in the gland itself, but the cells and neuralgia suggest a secretory function. Removal of the pineal or injection of extracts have demonstrated a definite effect on sexual function, particularly in birds and rats. The pineal takes up relatively large amounts of the amino acid, tryptophan, and synthesizes it into a variety of indoles:

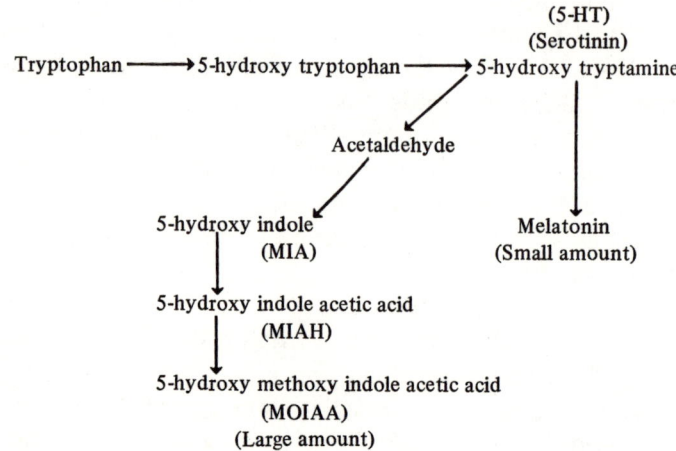

NEUROHYPOPHYSIS AND OTHER HORMONAL AGENTS 81

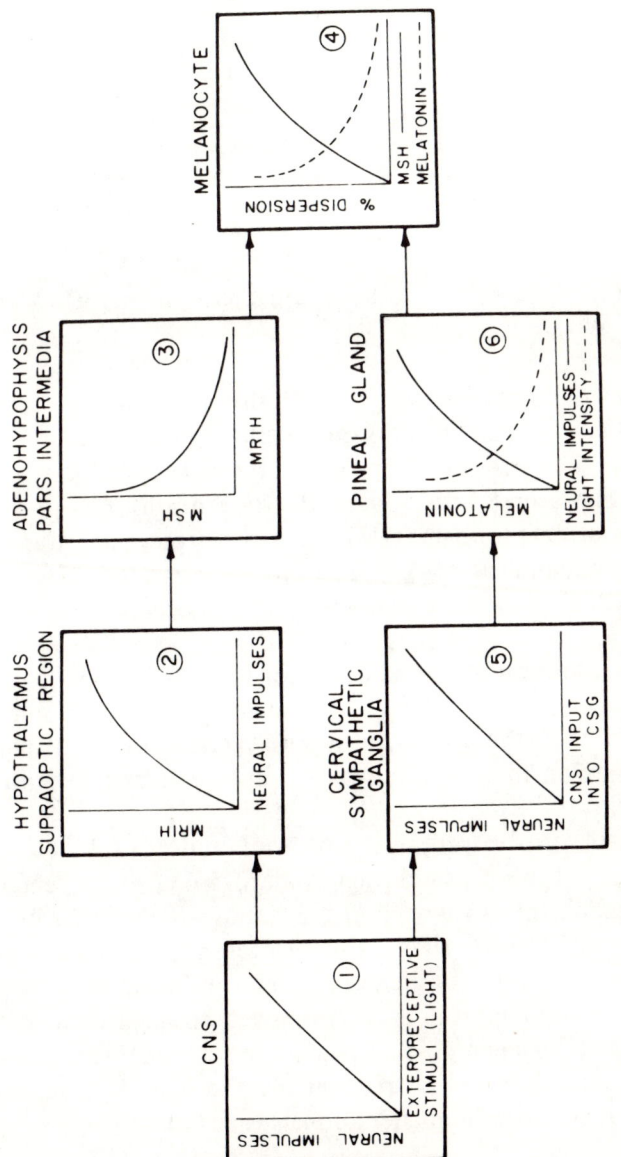

Figure 5.6. Control of the pineal gland indicating the numerous nervous connections that enter into the control. (From J. Kline, *Biological Foundation of Biomedical Engineering*, Little, Brown, Boston, 1976, with permission.)

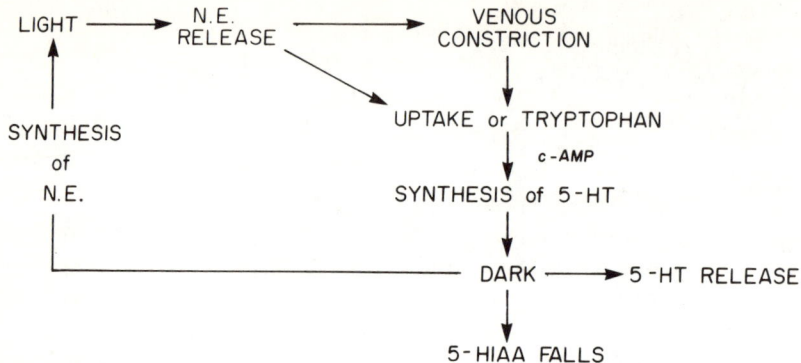

Figure 5.7. The synthesis of 5-hydroxy tryptophan in the pineal under the influence of light.

The pineal is almost unique in the rhythmicity and high amplitude of its circadian rhythm. The rhythm is triggered by light—or perhaps by dark—and the peak secretion of the *glandular* products occurs at midnight. The secretion is apparently triggered by norepinephrine. The 5-hydroxy tryptophan (5-HT) is high in the gland during daylight and is released at night. The circadian rhythm continues in the blind animal, indicating that sight is not necessary for the light-dark reaction.

The exact function of the pineal is not well established, and which of its components is the actual hormone has not been elucidated. It is interesting that the gland produces a variety of small peptides, which are similar in structure to the hypothalamic sex-inhibiting hormones.

The control of the pineal is not well understood because the feedback has not been established (Figure 5.6). It is clear that in light, norepinephrine is released at the gland, which causes uptake of trypotophan at receptor sites. In the presence of c-AMP, 5-HT is synthesized and stored. In the dark, 5-HT is released by some neural stimuli, and norepinephrine is resynthesized to begin to cycle again (Figure 5.7). It has been postulated that the seasonal sex variation in birds and mammals may be triggered by the light-dark response of the pineal. Its function in higher animals is not clear.

THE PROSTAGLANDINS

Within the last 10 years, a class of 20-hydroxy unsaturated fatty acids have been implicated in a wide variety of physiological processes. In fact, with the possible exception of c-AMP, the prostaglandins (PG) have an almost ubiquitous distribution. The prostaglandins are related to the pentaenoic, arachidonic, and trienoic essential fatty acids. There are some 15 derivatives of at least six primary prostaglandins all derived from the 20-carbon basic compound. There are two major types of prostaglandins, PGE and PGF, which are isomerically different and not interchangeable. The major difference is that PGE has a ketone on position 9 in the ring structure (Figure 5.8), while PGF has a hydroxyl group on the same carbon.

The prostaglandins can be synthesized by a wide variety of tissues in their microsomal system. Theophylline, which potentiates the action of c-AMP, also potentiates the action of PGE, implicating c-AMP in the process. The prostaglandins are destroyed rapidly in many tissues, particularly in the lung. A major problem in understanding the physiology of the prostaglandins has been the apparently contradictory results that have been obtained. Actually, it now appears that PGE and PGF can produce opposed activities in the same tissue. PGF, for example, causes the fallopian tube to relax while PGE increases motility.

Although the prostaglandins have many effects, the major line of investigation has been on sexual function ever since von Euler found prostaglandins in sperm. PGE has several diverse activities on the female reproductive tract: it causes contraction of the pregnant uterus when instilled, and it has been widely used as an abortifacient. It also appears in high concentration during the latter stages of pregnancy and may stimulate parturition.

PGE also mimics the action of LH by stimulating progesterone production in the corpus luteum. LH is not necessary for progesterone production in the presence of PGE. On the other hand,

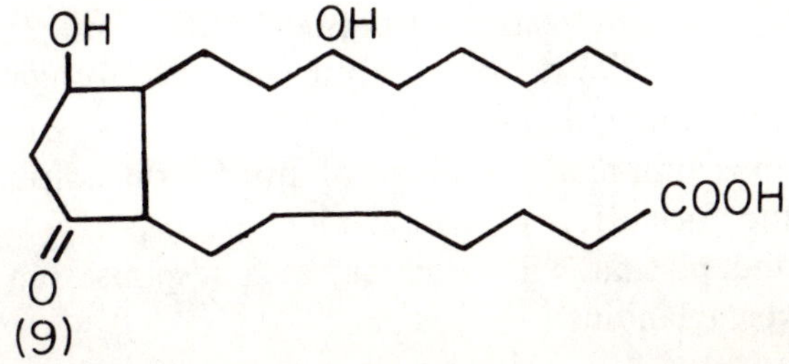

Figure 5.8. A generalized structure of the prostaglandins.

PGF is luteolytic in the same system, apparently by inhibiting LH production. In some species, the presence of LTH or estrogen will block the activity of PGF, indicating that PGF may operate at the hypothalamic feedback level. There must also be a direct action of PGF on ovarian receptors because PGF is active in the hypophysectomized animal given LTH. The situation regarding the site of action is not totally clear. If pentabarbital is given to an animal at the proper time, LTH secretion is blocked, and LH is not released. In such an animal, PGE will release LH and cause ovulation. PGF causes intense venous constriction in the ovary and uterus; this decrease in blood supply has been proposed as the luteolytic initiating factor. It is known that the developed endometrium produces PGE, which apparently then constricts the ovarian arteries to cause hyporemia.

The rupture of the follicle at ovulation has been tied to PGE; it does not rupture properly in the absence of prostaglandins. PGE may be necessary for LRF to release LH from the pituitary. Interestingly, the formation of prostaglandins is stimulated by LH, indicating a positive feedback. On the other hand, if the corpus luteum is functional and secreting progesterone and estrogen, PGE will block steroidogenesis. This may be the way in which function of the corpus luteum is halted at each menstrual cycle and during pregnancy. In the menstrual cycle, PGE may stimulate corpus luteum formation and LH production when the body begins to secrete. The high PGE may eventually block secretion, and thus the corpus luteum becomes nonfunctional.

Analogs have been developed to the prostaglandins in order to make them more readily available. The 17-oxy-13 prostynoic acid is a prostaglandin-blocker, whereas other derivatives are longer acting and more powerful than the parent compounds. In males, the prostaglandins have been implicated in enhancement of sperm motility and androgen production, but the effects are not clear.

One of the most interesting effects of PGE is on adipose tissue. Prostaglandins will inhibit the lipolysis usually brought about by ACTH, glucagon, and epinephrine.

Prostaglandins mimic the actions of insulin on adipose tissue in stimulating the formation of triglycerides from NEFA. High levels of FFA in the plasma will produce, as a response, an immediate increase in prostaglandins.

Indomethacin has also been found to block the biosynthesis of prostaglandins. Prostaglandin production is strongly inhibited by aspirin. Some observers believe this causes the antiinflammatory action of aspirin, which correlates well with observations that prostaglandins cause inflammatory reaction such as wheals and flares upon subdermal injection.

PGE and PGF have potent circulatory effects. Usually, the effects are opposite to each other, i.e., PGE causes vasoconstriction in lung and kidney blood vessels whereas PGF causes dilation in the same vessels. However, in the kidney, the vasoconstrictor effect may be of greater interest because PGE initiates the liberation of renin from the kidney, and higher concentrations of PGE appear in renal hypertension, which may be caused by the renin-angiotension mechanism. PGE also effects sympathetic amino actions. When renal vasoconstriction is initiated by norepinephrine, PG is released within a few minutes to cause vasodilation and diuresis.

The aforementioned relationships between the prostaglandins and c-AMP may partially explain the widespread activity of prostaglandins in many tissues. It is surprising that a substance with so many activities should have been investigated only in the last 20 years. The final story has not yet been written.

References

Chard, T. "Recent Trends in the Physiology of the Posterior Pituitary." *Current Topics in Exper. Endocrin.* 1 (1971): 81-120.

Dousa, T. P. "Role of Cyclic AMP in the Action of Anti-Diuretic Hormones on Kidney." *Life Sciences* 13 (1973): 1033-1040.

Kent, C. and M. A. Williams, "The Nature of the Hypothalamo-Neurophypophysial Neurosecretion in the Rat." *Journal of Cell Physiology* 60 (1974): 554-570.

Ganong, W. F. and I. Martini. *Frontiers in Neuroendocrinology.* New York: Oxford University Press, 1973.

Leaf, A. and C. H. Coggins, "The Neurohypophysis." In R. H. Williams, *Textbook of Endocrinology*, 5th ed. Baltimore: Williams & Wilkins, 1974.

Quay, W. B. *Pineal Chemistry*, Springfield: Charles C Thomas, 1974.

Swabb, D. F. "The Hypothalamo-Neurohypophysial System and Reproduction." *Prog. Brain Res.* 38 (1972): 225-224.

The following review articles cover most of the details about the prostaglandins and provide a wealth of references.

Hinman, J. W. "Prostaglandins." *Am. Rev. of Biochem.* **41** (1972): 161.
Pharris, B. B. and J. E. Shaw. "Prostaglandins in Reproduction." *Ann. Rev. of Physiol.* **36** (1974): 391.
Weeks, J. R. "Prostaglandins." *Ann. Rev. of Pharm.* **12** (1972): 317.

6
The Thyroid

The thyroid has been known from the days of antiquity; the gland was described by the Greek physician Galen and given its name in 1656 by Thomas Wharton. The principal hormone was isolated a few years ago by Kendall, and real progress in understanding thyroid physiology has been made only in the last 20 years.

The thyroid consists of two separate lobes lying on either side of the trachea below the larynx. The blood supply is profuse. The gland itself is composed of follicles containing a proteinlike material, the colloid, surrounded by a single layer of epithelial cells (Figure 6.1).

Any single follicle seems to function as a coordinated unit, since all of its cells appear to be in the same state of activity, whereas adjacent follicles may vary widely in secretory function. The thyroid is the outstanding example of an endocrine organ that does not store the products of secretion within the cells of the organ. The thyroid hormone may be either secreted directly into the bloodstream or stored within the follicular fluid, with the latter method predominating.

The thyroid histology is related to its function. Cell size changes markedly with activity of the gland; during hyperactivity, the cells become columnar in appearance as distinguished from the more cuboidal cell type of the normal quiescent gland. The size and number of mitochondria in the follicular cells are greater during periods of thyroid activity, and less during periods of relative inactivity. A pro-

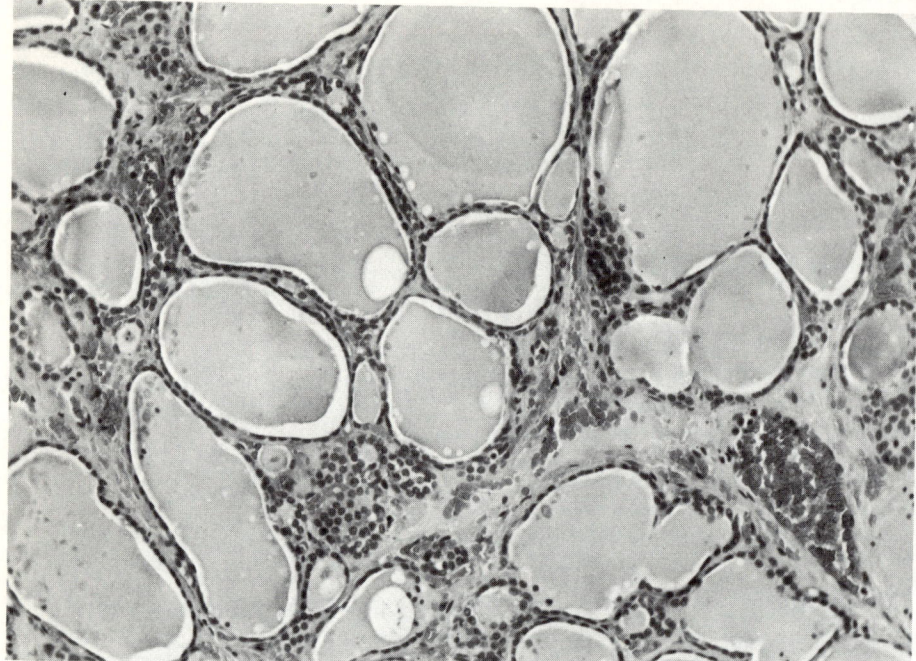

Figure 6.1. Microscopic photo of the thyroid follicles showing clearly the large colloid-filled follicle surrounded by the columnar epithelium of the thyroid cells.

teolytic enzyme, that appears to be necessary for the release of hormone from the colloid is also increased during activity and decreased during rest.

IODINE METABOLISM

As will be seen later, the most characteristic constituent of the thyroid hormone is the element iodine. In order to appreciate some of the relationships of the thyroid to other metabolic processes, it is necessary to consider some of the aspects of iodine metabolism.

Iodine enters the body in the diet (Figure 6.2) either as the iodide (iodate, etc.) ion or in organic form. It is absorbed rapidly from the gut into the plasma. The blood inorganic iodide, which is either unbound or very loosely bound to plasma proteins, reaches the thyroid gland via its blood supply. Iodide is taken up so rapidly that it is

THE THYROID

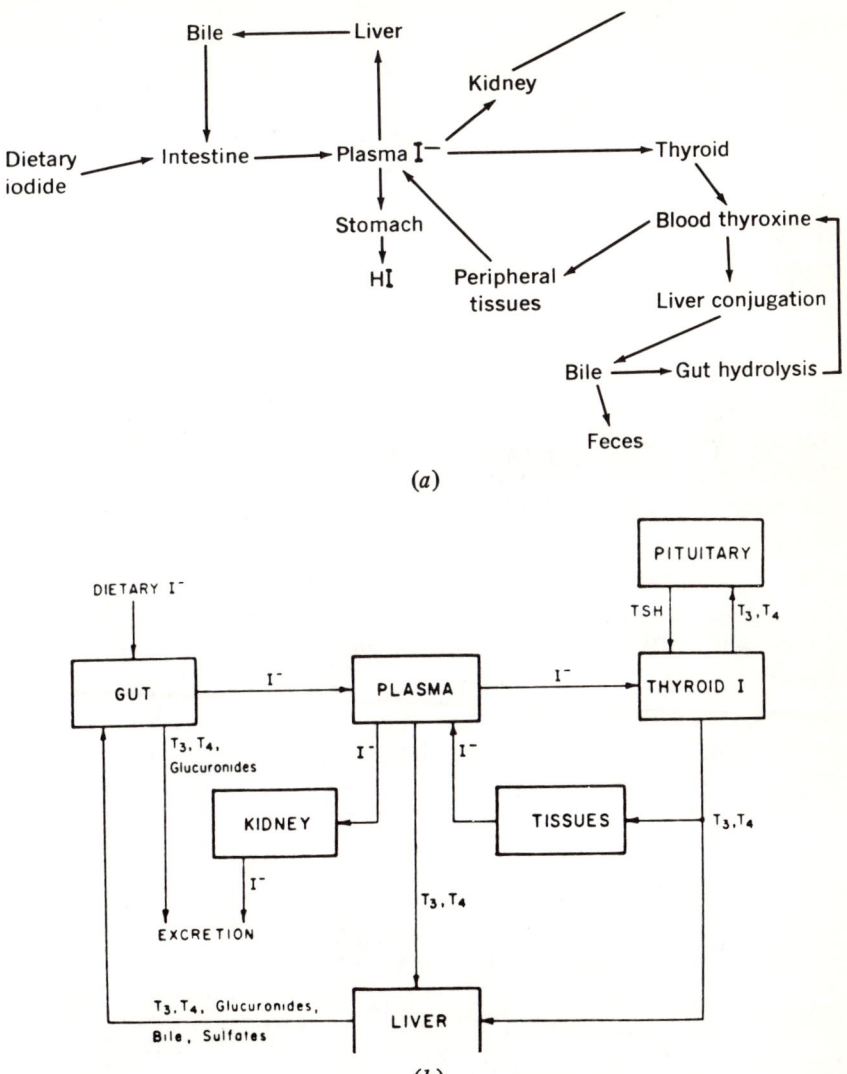

Figure 6.2. (a) The circulation of iodine in the body illustrating the paths that return it to the general circulation as a measure of conservation. (b) A simple control diagram illustrating the same facts as (a) in an exchange system.

often said to be *trapped* although the term *pumped* is preferred by some, in order to emphasize the intracellular concentrating ability of the gland. This is a stage that is independent of further glandular activity or synthesis of hormone, provided enough iodine is obtained.

There is considerable excretion of iodide by the kidney. Clearance of iodide varies with its concentration in plasma. The normal iodide clearance is about 31 milliliters/minute, but in iodide deficiency this can be decreased to about 0.05 milliliters per minute. The iodide ion appears to be handled by the kidney in a manner similar to chloride. In addition to the ingested iodide, there is also iodide in the body that results from the degradation of thyroid hormones and precursors. On a low iodine intake, this released iodine is an important component of the iodine pool available to the thyroid gland. Some of the iodine is also secreted as hydrogen iodine in place of hydrochloric acid by the chief cells of the stomach.

The administration of large amounts of iodide will lead to saturation of the trapping mechanism of the thyroid with a decreased uptake of iodine. This does not, however, usually lead to any detectable increase in the amounts of stored or secreted thyroid hormone. In contrast, when the supply of inorganic iodide is low, the first change is an increase in the iodide-retention capacity of the thyroid. There is an increased turnover of thyroxine, but not a quantitative deficiency. The gland undergoes hypertrophy and hyperplasia. Eventually, failure may occur, and characteristic signs of thyroid deficiency develop. Figure 6.3 outlines the daily turnover of iodine in the tissues. The most interesting observation is the large store of

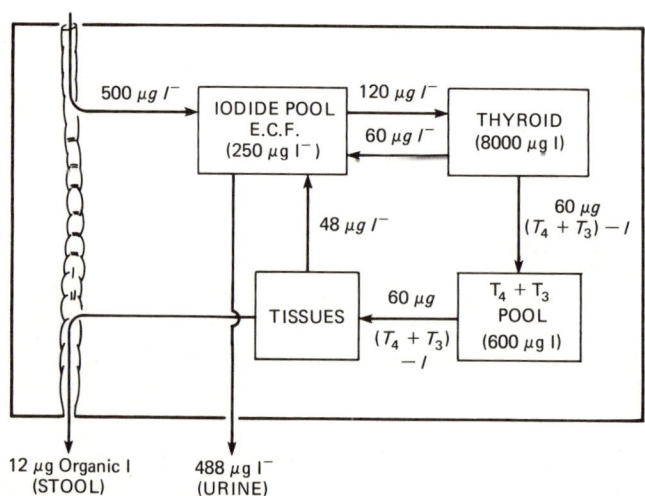

Figure 6.3. The volumes of distribution of iodine in the circulating pool. Note the relatively small amount of circulating thyroid hormone.

iodine in the thyroid gland. This obviously serves as a buffer to sudden changes in iodine input. The other interesting phase of the diagram is the relatively small amount—actually micrograms—of iodine present in the active hormones triiodothyronine (T_3) and thyroxine (T_4).

The ready physical combination of iodine with other materials, especially protein, has led to the concept that some thyroid hormone might be synthesized in extrathyroidal tissues, especially since the combination is apparently a simple mass-action relationship. The uptake of iodine by the thyroid, on the other hand, must be due to specific metabolic activity, since the concentration of iodine in the thyroid can become many time higher than that of other tissues. The ratio of thyroid iodide to blood serum iodide (*T/S ratio*) often is greater than 100.

When circulating iodine is trapped by the thyroid gland, it can be readily synthesized into the thyroid hormone (Figure 6.4). If the process of synthesis is blocked by an antithyroid compound such as thiouracil, the uptake of iodine can continue for only a few hours. If the blocking drug had been administered for several days previous to the iodine-uptake test, the greater vascularity often resulting from

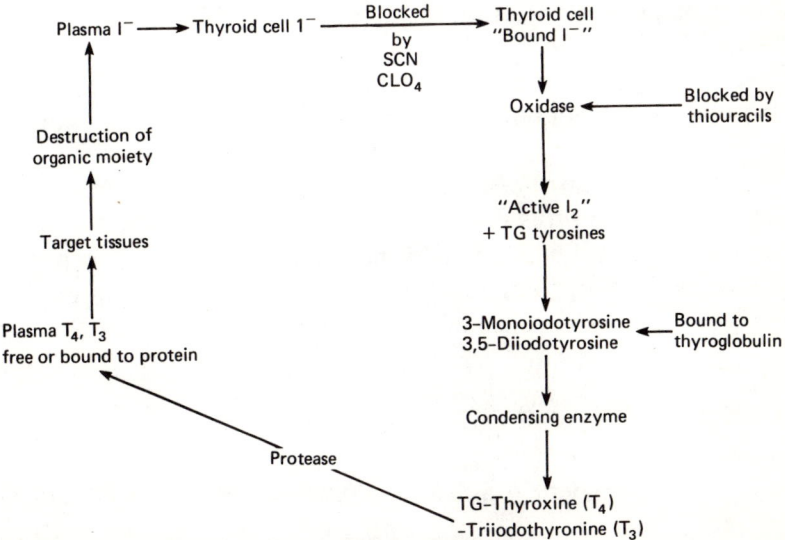

Figure 6.4. A general scheme of thyroid hormone formation indicating the points at which synthesis can be blocked by specific inhibitors.

the hyperplasia will produce increased apparent iodine uptake on a temporary basis. The amount of iodine that can be taken up under these circumstances is said to represent the *iodide space* of the gland. The circulation of iodine is fortunately a simple matter to measure, for the element can be readily and cheaply obtained in the radioactive form I^{131} and I^{125} in a high degree of purity. It is also possible to measure the nonradioactive I^{127} by its catalysis of the colorimetric oxidation-reduction reaction between ceric sulfate and arsenious acid.

Iodine occupying the iodide space is in a dynamic equilibrium with the blood. Higher blood levels of iodide increase the iodide space, but the effect is limited. The T/S ratio is relatively constant in the thiouracil-treated rat over wide ranges of iodine concentration indicating the nonmetabolic features of this form of uptake.

The uptake of radioactive iodide by the thyroid is increased by the thyrotrophic hormone (TSH). This is true whether the organic synthetic mechanism is blocked by thiouracil or not, although in this case the iodine cannot long be retained. It has been postulated that TSH increases the number of receptor sites for iodine uptake into the cells of the thyroid. The total activity (uptake) in the thyroid is determined by a balance between two factors: (1) the influence of TSH and low iodine concentration in the thyroid to increase uptake, and (2) some inhibitor, which tends to decrease the uptake. The inhibitor may be organically bound iodine since blocking of the formation of the organically bound form increases the uptake of the inorganic form.

The site of action of TSH in stimulating the thyroid gland is of interest. Two mechanisms suggest themselves. It is possible to increase either the equilibrium constant of enzymatic reactions, thus producing more product, or to increase the velocity but not the equilibrium. Some years ago, Michealis and Menten defined systems of this type as:

$$\text{Enzyme} + \text{Substrate} \underset{K_2}{\overset{K_1}{\rightleftarrows}} \text{Enzyme} - \text{Substrate Complex} \overset{K_3}{\rightarrow} \text{Product} + \text{Enzyme}$$

where the equilibrium in constant *Km* is

$$K_m = \frac{K_2 + K_3}{K_1}$$

and can be measured because at one-half the maximal reaction velocity, the velocity = K_m. With this technique, it can be demonstrated that TSH affects only velocity but not K_m, whereas competitive drugs affect K_m.

Because TSH is a protein, it probably acts through a second messenger (see p. 33); in fact, c-AMP is necessary for TSH action. When theophylline, which blocks phosphodiesterase, is administered, c-AMP is not as readily destroyed and TSH action is potentiated.

When synthesis of thyroid hormone is stimulated by TSH, the ratio of T_3 to T_4 changes. Under normal conditions, the T_3/T_4 ratio is about 0.20. Under intense stimulation, it may become four. The same phenomenon occurs in extreme iodine deficiency. It can be reasoned that the more active T_3 plus the 25 percent less iodine per molecule results in conservation of iodine.

In addition to the control of iodine uptake previously mentioned, perchlorate, thiocyanate, and, to some extent, the other halogens will block the iodide *pump*, thus preventing uptake of the inorganic iodide. Adequate doses of either perchlorate or thiocyanate cause the thyroid to release any inorganic iodide present. As a result, organification is indirectly depressed, although these compounds must be administered several times a day in order to maintain their action at a maximum.

The release of iodide by various agents as well as the rapid concentration of the ion in the thyroid suggests that it must be bound in a loose form that is readily dissociated. If binding did not occur to some extent, it would not be possible to obtain the occasional high T/S ratio of 200 or more. It has been suggested that cytochromes must be involved in some way in the complex that accomplishes the uptake and binding of the iodine, since both the iodide pump and the cytochromes are readily inhibited by specific ions and both are unaffected by thiouracil.

THE THYROID HORMONE

Depending upon the animal, most of the iodide trapped by the thyroid is synthesized into organic forms. Present evidence indicates that tyrosine present in the thyroglobulin protein molecule is iodinated, first to monoiodotyrosine, then to diiodotyrosine (Figure 6.5). Two molecules of iodotyrosine are then combined oxidatively, with the elimination of alanine side-chain, to form an iodo-diphenyl ether-

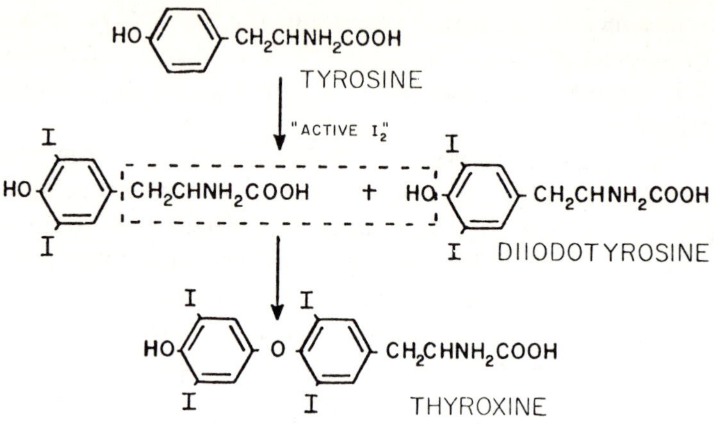

94 INTEGRATION AND COORDINATION OF METABOLIC PROCESSES

$$HO-C_6H_4-CH_2CHNH_2COOH \quad \text{TYROSINE}$$

$$\downarrow \text{"ACTIVE } I_2^{"}$$

$$I\text{-}HO\text{-}C_6H_3(I)\text{-}CH_2CHNH_2COOH \quad + \quad HO\text{-}C_6H_3(I)\text{-}CH_2CHNH_2COOH \quad \text{DIIODOTYROSINE}$$

$$\downarrow$$

$$HO\text{-}C_6H_2(I_2)\text{-}O\text{-}C_6H_3(I)\text{-}CH_2CHNH_2COOH \quad \text{THYROXINE}$$

Figure 6.5. The formation of two molecules of diiodotyrosine, which are then combined with elimination of one alanine side-chain to yield thyroxine. Although not so shown, all amino acids are doubly linked by peptide bonds involving the amino and carboxyl groups.

containing complex amino acid called an iodothyronine ("thyronine" is the name of the thyroxine molecule stripped of its four iodine atoms). Two diiodotyrosines combine to form thyroxine (T_4), quantitatively the major hormonally active material present. When one monoidotyrosine and one diiodotyrosine participate, much less of it is present than of thyroxine. It was believed that the tetraiodo form was the only active thyroid hormone, but when 3,5,3'-T_3 was discovered in 1952, it was found to be effective at a considerably lower dose level. The gland secretes about 85 percent T_4 and the remainder as T_3.

Organification of iodine should be considered as part of the overall process of iodine retention, since trapped iodine cannot long be held by the thyroid unless organic iodine is formed. In human beings, about 20 to 40 percent of an administered dose of radioactive iodide is normally found in the thyroid gland 24 hours later, but the higher figure may be attained in 4 hours by an overactive gland, indicating the increased rate of synthesis.

It must be realized that this synthesis results in formation of thyroxine and T_3 already in a peptide linkage integral within the thyroglobulin molecule. Ordinarily, none of this large molecular weight (670,000) protein escapes from the gland. As part of the TSH-maintained mechanism for release of thyroid hormone, proteolysis occurs, liberating iodotyrosines, as well as T_4, T_3, and other, noniodinated amino acids. Enzymatic deiodination of diiodotyrosines takes place within the gland, with the resulting iodine being reused by the gland's iodinating mechanism. Iodothyronines (T_4, T_3) are not deiodinated in the thyroid gland but are released to the bloodstream as free forms of the hormone. In the case of hyperthyroidism, the apparent demand on the gland is such that little hormone is stored. The normally low, cuboidal epithelial cells enlarge (hypertrophy) and may increase in number (hyperplasia) if hyperactivity continues. The nature of the stimulus to the gland is not known, but the histological picture is very similar to that seen in iodine deficiency. It has suggested that there is such an increased peripheral demand for thyroxine that the thyroid gland is unable to obtain enough iodine for organification in significant excess of demand. There is no known basis for the accelerated thyroxine need, and many researchers still prefer an explanation of increased TSH secretion, even though insufficient direct data exist to demonstrate elevated blood levels of this trophic hormone. The presence of long-acting thyroid-stimulator globulin (LATS), of nonpituitary origin, in the blood plasma of thyrotoxic patients offers a possible resolution of these discrepancies.

The Circulating Thyroid Hormone. It is generally agreed that thyroxine is the principal element of circulating thyroid hormone, with smaller amounts of 3,5,3'-triiodothyronine also being present. Thyroxine is nearly all bound to plasma protein, although a small amount must be free to diffuse into tissue cells. For several years, this binding was believed to be exclusively to globulin (TBG), but a protein (prealbumin) (TBPA) with electropheretic mobility greater than albumin in some buffers has been implicated. Since electrophoresis must be carried out under conditions different from those existing *in vivo*, it is difficult to decide at present the exact details of physiological transport. It is important to realize that such a binding is quite different from that employed in the well-known chemical evaluation of hormonal iodine in the blood plasma, the "protein-bound iodine" (PBI). For this determination, plasma (or serum) proteins are precipitated, carrying down both T_4 and T_3 in coprecipitated form.

An understanding of the exact relationship of T_3 and T_4 to the protein pool is essential if the physiology of the gland is to be understood. The thyroid gland secretes about 85 percent T_4 and 15 percent T_3. In the tissues, and before it performs metabolic activity, about 40 percent of the T_4 is converted to T_3.

$$T_4 + TBP \rightleftharpoons T_4\,TBP \longrightarrow T_3 + TBP \rightleftharpoons T_3\,TBP$$

$$\frac{T_4}{T_4\,TBP} = 1/K_{T_4} = 99.97\% \text{ bound} = 2 \text{ Ng\%}$$

$$\frac{T_3}{T_3\,TBP} = 1/K = 99.70\% \text{ bound} = 4 \text{ Ng\%}$$

Although T_3 and T_4 are almost totally bound, it must be clear that T_3 still has 30 times the free concentration of T_4. As *all* of the activity of thyroid hormone can be attributed only to the *free* form, T_3 is much more active metabolically.

The hormones are bound to globulin, and T_4 is bound to prealbumin as well. The binding *capacity* is 200 Ngm% (nanograms per cent) T_4 to TBG and 1,500 Ngm% to TBPA, while T_3 has TBG with a capacity of 160 Ngm%.

The relationship of these proteins to the thyroid activity is important. If for any reason the TBG falls (as in starvation), not as much can be bound, and the *free* T_3 and T_4 rises. Demands of the tissues, decreased secretion of TSH through feedback, and the equilibrium constant returns the free thyroid hormone to essentially normal levels but with decreased storage-and-transport facilities. On the other hand, when TBG increases (as in pregnancy), more T_3 and T_4 are bound, the free concentration decreases, and more TSH is secreted to restore the free level to normal. The critical point arises in clinical studies where the PBI, which is essentially the TBG, is measured as an indication of thyroid function. It should be apparent that perfectly normal thyroid function can occur with abnormal TBGs.

The binding of thyroid hormones by protein is highly specific. Other isomers and similar hormones do not bind as well. T_3 is not as tightly bound as T_4. There are other differences in T_4 and T_3. The T_3 space in the liver is about 30 percent of the total distribution, while T_4 space in the liver is only 6 percent of its distribution. As a result, there is a much larger pool of T_3.

Measurement of the half-life indicates that T_3 has a half-life of 1 day whereas the half-life of T_4 is about 6 days.

Each of these facts indicate that T_3 may be more active than T_4; in fact, the overall effect is such that T_3 is about three times as active in the human as T_4. In fact, some investigators believe T_4 is relatively inactive. It is true that T_4 does not stimulate nuclear activity and mitochrondia nearly as well as T_3.

Analogs have been developed that block the action of thyroid hormones by binding to cellular receptors. These receptors apparently have two loci of action, a binding function and a functional group. Thyroid analogs that block the usual thyroid hormone action apparently can block binding but do not combine with the functional group.

By the same type of investigation, it is possible to separate the calorigenic action of hormones and the thyroid-stimulating (goiter-preventing) action. Analogs have been produced that vary 100 times in these properties.

Metabolism of Thyroid Hormones. Thyroxine can be broken down by many tissues, including some that do not respond metabolically to injection of the hormone, such as the brain. The rate of turnover of T_4 is slow, with a half-life in humans of about 6 days, whereas that for T_3 is about 1 day. The net result of tissue metabolism of T_4 and T_3 is the production of iodide, which reenters the circulation and is partly lost in the urine, partly recaptured by the thyroid gland. The body probably breaks down about 200 micrograms of thyroxine replace the loss. Actually, it is estimated that 15 micrograms of iodide suffice to supply the daily bodily requirements, demonstrating the extent of conservation of the element. About 10 milligrams of organic iodine are stored in the thyroid. On this basis, the daily turnover of iodine represents only about 1 percent of the available hormone. The combination of this reserve and the recirculation of iodide are protective mechanisms, and long periods of iodine deprivation can occur before signs of deficiency develop.

As would be expected, the alanine side-chain of T_4 and T_3 is susceptible to attack by deamination plus decarboxylation to produce the corresponding iodothyroacetic acid derivatives. These compounds have been identified from both *in vivo* and *in vitro* chemical alterations of thyroid hormones. At one time, they were considered to display unusual metabolic activities, but it has since been realized that they are only about 15 percent as active as the respective parent compound. The iodothyroacetic acids can also be deiodinated by many tissues.

Control of Thyroid Secretion. In brief summary, it is apparent that the control of hormone secretion is under the influence of TSH from the anterior pituitary as modified by the hypothalamus. Evidence is available that TSH secretion is influenced by the circulating thyroid hormone concentration. Injection of thyroxine directly into the pituitary that has been severed from nervous connections results in the inhibition of TSH production. The uptake of radioiodine by the pituitary is exceeded only by that of the thyroid and of the gut, although the significance of this finding is not clear. Thyroid uptake of iodine is controlled by the pituitary release of TSH. Hypophysectomy results in a marked decrease in uptake (about 10 percent of the injected dose) as compared to normal (30 percent) or to animals given TSH (60 percent). It has been claimed that some regulation is exerted by the thyroid itself, since *in vitro* incubation of thyroid tissue with TSH results in inactivation of the thyrotrophin. In some cases of hyperthyroidism, it has been suggested that the hyperactive thyroid destroys the TSH as rapidly as it is produced so that no feedback occurs and continuous stimulation by the pituitary is the final result. Removal of the thyroid causes the formation of typical "thyroidectomy" cells in the pituitary.

TSH has a direct influence upon the thyroid, causing increased oxygen consumption, increased amounts of proteolytic enzymes, increased number of intracellular droplets, increased height and size of thyroid cells, and increase in size and weight of the gland. The increase in cell height brought about by TSH administration is one of the most common bases for quantitative estimations of TSH activity. Conversely, in the absence of TSH, there is a markedly decreased cell height, decrease in weight of the gland, and decreases in other evidences of functional activity. These facts are summarized in Figure 6.6.

Figure 6.6 is a diagram of the plasmaprotein binding which has already been discussed. Figure 6.7 demonstrates clearly the many possible feedback mechanisms in the thyroid and the many questionable points that have not yet been fully explained. Both diagrams

THE THYROID 99

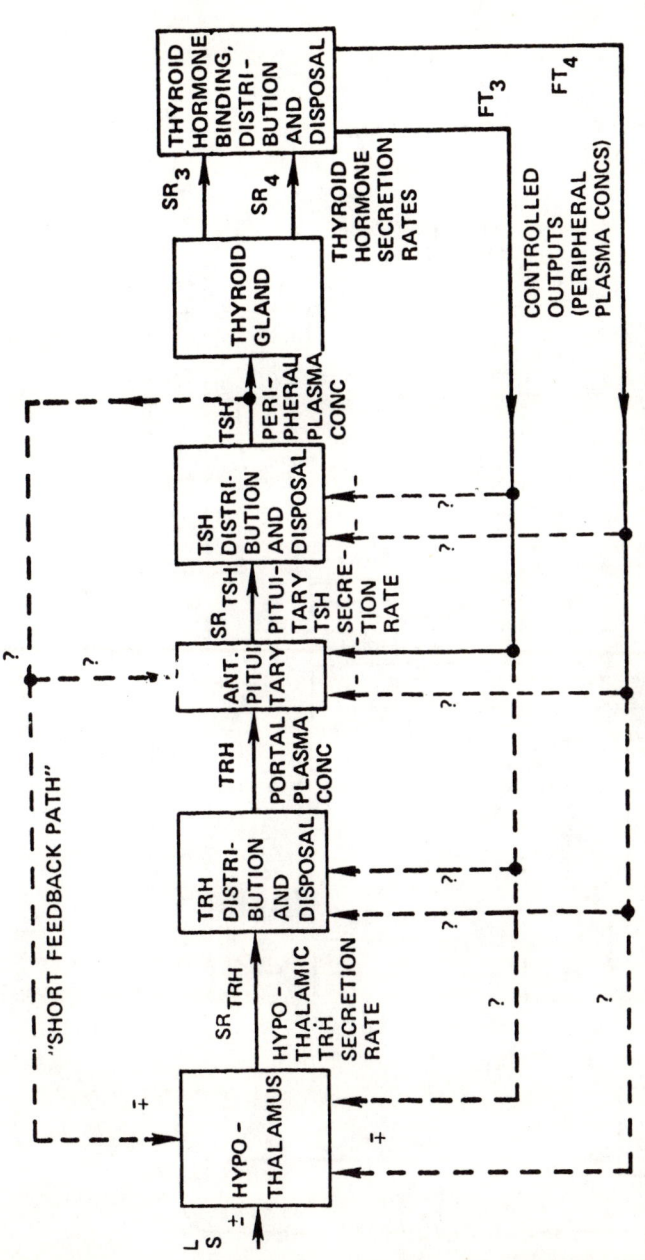

Figure 6.6 The regulation of thyroid secretion, taking into account the distribution as well as the normal feedback. (Courtesy of Dr. Joseph Di Stefano.)

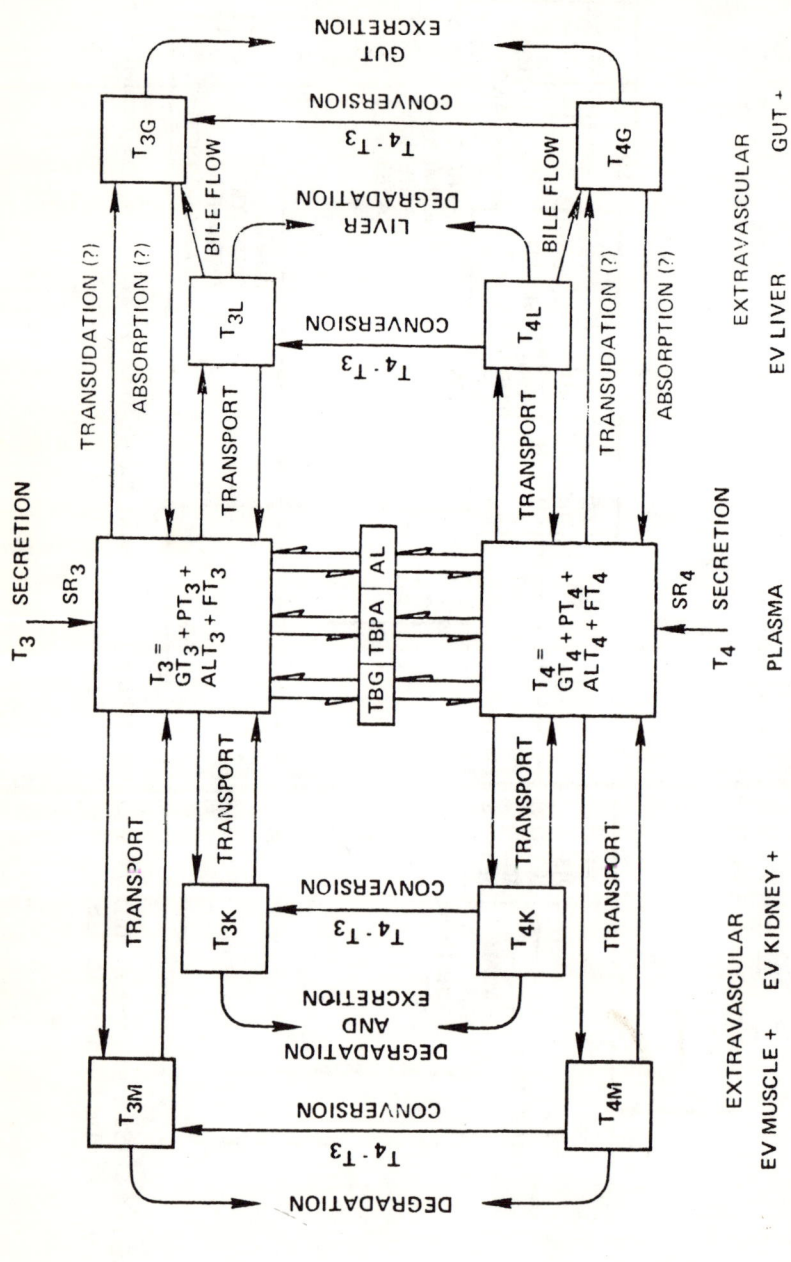

Figure 6.7. Another view of the data on thyroid function, illustrating the binding of thyroxine as explained in the text. (Courtesy of Dr. Joseph Di Stefano.)

indicate the distribution of T_3 and T_4 in tissues and between albumin and globulin in the plasma.

ACTIVITY OF THE THYROID HORMONE

The thyroid secretes a general metabolic hormone. It is able to increase the oxygen uptake of tissues and to increase the general metabolic rate. As a result, it is not surprising that the thyroid has effects on many tissues and on many processes.

The thyroid exerts both a fine and a coarse control on metabolism. Thyroid hormone when first administered produces an immediate fine control, an adjustment in the specific activity of enzyme systems. By 2 or 3 days later, a coarse control exemplified by the synthesis of new oxidative enzymes begins to appear. Figure 6.8 gives an indication of the time span of the various processes, ranging from minutes to days for the complete process to occur.

Thyroid hormone can be said to have a "permissive" action in much the same way as adrenal steroids. Many processes in growth and maturation and many metabolic processes do not go well without the hormone, whereas relatively small amounts permit an immediate response. Speculation has centered around the ability of the hormone to increase c-AMP, which can then serve as the second messenger for other hormones.

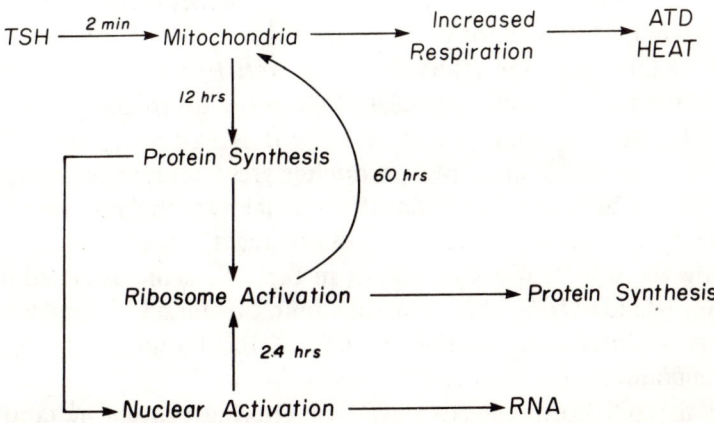

Figure 6.8. The activation times for the various processes by which TSH activates the thyroid gland.

One of the major effects of thyroid hormone is the calorigenic action and the increase in oxygen consumption that follows its administration. In a sense, this occurs because the processes of energy production become less efficient. Oxygen is usually coupled to the electron-transport system in the cell, so that there is a constant ratio between ATP produced and oxygen consumed (P/O ratio). The P/O ratio is about 3.0 (theoretical). When thyroid hormone is administered, the processes are said to become "uncoupled" and the ratio P/O $<$ 3. In a real sense, the cell "spins its wheels" and consumes more oxygen in less efficient processes.

The tissues comprising the bulk of the body weight (skeletal muscle, liver, kidney, heart) respond to thyroxine injection with increased oxygen uptake. In contrast, no effect is shown by the thyroid itself, nerve tissue, gonads, and accessory reproductive structures of both sexes, spleen, and gastrointestinal smooth muscle. Consistent increases result only upon *in vivo* administration of hormone, and most reports of *in vitro* action have been unconvincing. This may be due to the long latent period of the hormone, even in the case of T_3, which may be required to synthesize extra oxidative enzymes and precursors, so that such processes cannot occur in the usual time period of an *in vitro* experiment.

Storage of kidney and liver tissue slices at a low temperature (5° C) permits survival for several days and a clear demonstration of a delayed *in vitro* T_4 effect on oxygen consumption. Attempts to show that this latent period is required for production of an especially active form of T_4 have not been successful.

The metabolic action (the *calorigenic activity*) is greater in young animals than in old and is greatest of all in the thyroidectomized animal. The hypothyroid animal or patient is extremely sensitive to thyroid, with small amounts producing great effects on metabolic rates. It has been suggested that the normal hypothalamus-pituitary-thyroid system in some way removes or inactivates thyroxine, thus reducing the effect of a given dose; in fact, T_3 is metabolized in the pituitary gland. It is also probable that the target tissues become sensitive to thyroxine in the absence of the hormone, a principle often encountered in endocrinology.

The thyroid hormone is capable of altering protein metabolism. In hypothyroidism, the young individual fails to grow and muscular development is inadequate. It is probable that the processes of nitrogen metabolism are conditioned by the thyroid, and a certain level of thyroid activity is necessary to obtain maximum anabolic activity from growth hormone. On the other hand, large amounts of thyroxine increase the demand of the body for energy sources, increased gluconeogenesis results in extensive protein catabolism, and loss of weight is characteristic.

Somewhat similar effects could be predicted on carbohydrate metabolism. Excess thyroid hormone will tend to increase *glycogenolysis*, the breakdown of glycogen to supply the extra glucose needed for the increased metabolic functions. This results in decreased liver glycogen. In addition, thyroid hormone supplies additional glucose to the metabolic pool by increasing gluconeogenesis. The depressed gluconeogenesis seen in hypophysectomized animals can be reversed by T_4 administration although not quantitatively to the same extent as by the glucocorticoids. Together with the metabolic processes, which tend to increase the size of the glucose pool, the thyroid hormone increases the rate of absorption of glucose and other sugars from the intestine. Since glucose is a prime foodstuff, the most obvious explanation is that this action of thyroxine occurs simply because of the increased demand for energy sources.

Thyroxine exerts a definite effect on water and electrolytes. Excess thyroid will lead to the excretion of calcium and demineralization of bone. On the other hand, lack of thyroid will prevent the formation of normal bone by interfering with synthesis of the organic matrix. Optimal amounts of thyroid result in the laying-down, differentiation, and maturation of bone. In the thyroidectomized animal, the extracellular water compartment is increased in size, and administration of thyroid hormone results in prompt diuresis and sodium excretion. This is at least partly dependent upon mobilization of the subcutaneous edema fluid, which is so characteristic of thyroid-deficient individuals that it is the basis for the term *myxedema*.

Inadequate thyroid secretion in the young results in interference with development as well as failure of growth. The lack of differentiation of tissues is particularly well shown in the tadpole, which does not metamorphose if the thyroid is removed. Despite the reported failure of thyroxine to induce increased metabolism in the brain, the hypothyroid individual is dull. This can be corrected by thyroid hormone only if the deficiency occurred after the first few years of life, again illustrating the specific importance of thyroxine in promoting differentiation and development in the young animal.

As a result of its generalized metabolic activity, the thyroid would be expected to influence fat metabolism. Turnover of fat is increased, fat is mobilized from deposits, and cholesterol metabolism is increased under continued administration of thyroid hormone. Peripheral destruction of cholesterol is accelerated over hepatic production, resulting in a lowered plasma level. These effects are reversed in hypothyroidism, with destruction and excretion being so low that plasma cholesterol is increased.

The administration of excessive secretion of thyroid hormone increases blood pressure and heart rate, and continuation may lead to "high output" failure of the circulation. The heart production of the thyrotoxic is increased, and this, in turn, may lead to peripheral vasodilation (flushing) and temperature sensitivity. Although sluggish reactions of the hypothyroid individual are quickened upon hormonal treatment, one encounters nonspecific hyperactivity in the thyrotoxic animal. The myriad activities of the thyroid are summarized in Table 6.1.

Patients may display the enlargement of the gland known as *goiter*, which results from growth of the gland under stimulation of

Table 6.1. Activities of the thyroid.

Observed	Hypothyroid	Hyperthyroid
Behavior	Metabolism low, causes retardation	Metabolism high, nervousness
Growth	Decreased because metabolic material not available	Decreased because materials are burned up
Cardiovascular system	Decreased function because of low metabolism	Increased because of stimulation
Muscle	Weak because metabolic products not available	Weak because metabolic products are exhausted
Enzymes	Decreased activity	Increased activity
Carbohydrate metabolism	Slightly low blood sugar. Slow synthesis	Decreased blood sugar because of utilization
Fat metabolism	Increased fat in blood, liver, etc., because metabolism is decreased. Weight increase	T_4 stimulator FFA formation from fat to provide energy
Protein metabolism	Slightly negative nitrogen balance-permissive action	Nitrogen excretion, protein catabolism

larger than normal amounts of pituitary TSH. The first type of goiter arises in response to iodine deficiency, either absolute or relative. A geographic distribution of goiter, particularly in areas remote from seawater with its appreciable iodine content, has long been appreciated. Many of these regions of endemic goiter seem to be caused by the presence of specific goitrogens in certain vegetables. Even when the diet contains the usual amount of iodide, a long period of stress, such as adolescence, pregnancy, or continued exposure to cold, may increase the body's thyroid hormone needs beyond the availability of iodine, and thyroid enlargement occurs. *Colloid goiter*, in which there may be masses of large follicles distended with colloid, often results when a person with previous iodine deficiency returns to an adequate supply of the element.

ANTITHYROID DRUGS

As already mentioned, the iodide trap can be blocked by drugs such as thiocyanate and perchlorate, as well as by large amounts of iodide. An even wider variety of organic compounds has been found to inhibit production of organic iodine. Among the most potent are thiourea and its cyclic derivatives, such as thiouracil, 6-n-propylthiouracil, and methylmercaptoimidazole. These drugs are often employed to decrease the hyperactive thyroid gland, which is seen as part of the thyrotoxic syndrome. The thiobarbiturates such as thiopental and thioamylal, although ultra-short-acting as anesthetic barbiturates, are also thioureas and are capable of completely interrupting organification for many hours. Other compounds, such as the sulfas, hydroquinone, and so forth, are much less potent.

The only specific proposal as to the biochemical mechanisms for antithyroid action is that the thioureas compete with tyrosine for iodine activated by the glandular enzymes. In the final analysis, the success of the competition depends upon the relationship between the formation of "activated iodine" and the availability of the two types of iodine acceptors. Others have proposed inhibition of an iodide peroxidase, particularly to cover compounds not reacting readily with iodine.

For the first few days of administration of an antithyroid drug, the only detectable effect on gland function is a decreased I^{131} uptake; the iodine that is taken up can be discharged by perchlorate or thiocyanate, indicating its nonorganic nature. In fact, after prolonged feeding, all of the iodine in the gland may be present as inorganic iodide. As the supply of stored hormones is decreased, the signs and symptoms of hypothyroidism begin to develop. If the animal was previously normal, its thyroid undergoes tremendous enlargement, due first to cellular hypertrophy (low cuboidal changed to high columnar) and later to hyperplasia. This enlargement of the normal thyroid is the basis for the name of *goitrogen* applied to such chemical compounds. If the pituitary is removed, the hypertrophy and hyperplasia do not occur, pointing to TSH as the stimulus. Suppression of pituitary TSH can also be achieved by injecting T_4, T_3, or thyroactive materials. In fact, one procedure for the quantitative evaluation of thyroxine-like activity is by this antigoitrogenic action.

The action of thyroid-blocking agents such as propythiouracil is not a clear-cut inhibition of T_4 synthesis. It is now known that PTU also inhibits the conversion of T_4 to T_3 and may inhibit the action of T_4 and T_3 at the tissue level.

An interesting aspect of thyroid function is the report of high levels of T_3 and T_4 in some subjects. Apparently, the hormone cannot be utilized in peripheral tissues and so the concentration in plasma remains high. The indications are that this effect may be due to a lack of receptors in tissue cells.

The action of T_3 and T_4 in increasing cellular function can be explained on two theories. The number of mitochrondria can be increased, or the activity of each single unit can be increased. Present evidence indicates that the latter is the case.

THE THYROID AND OTHER ENDOCRINE ORGANS

There is an intimate relationship between the thyroid and the other endocrine organs, which would be expected from the known influence of the thyroid on cellular metabolism. The increased stress due to the greatly increased metabolism following thyroid administration leads to increased adrenocortical steroid output and hypertrophy of the gland. Decreased thyroid function is reflected in the gonads. In the female, the normal cyclic phenomena are interrupted; impairment of sperm production occurs in the male. Decreased sex drive might be due as much to the generally lowered metabolism as to any specific gonadal effects. Thyroid therapy is often undertaken for various complaints related to the reproductive function, especially in the human female, even in the absence of any objective evidence of hypothyroidism. The convenience of oral thyroid medication contributes to the frequency of this unjustified endocrine procedure.

It has been noted that cortisone administration will result in decreased I^{131} uptake, suggesting some effect of the adrenal on the thyroid. This is partly due to increased urinary loss of iodide, but it is also possible that the catabolic effect of the adrenal steroids prevents the laying down of colloid protein. In addition, corticoids inhibit ACTH production by the pituitary. Since TSH is presumably produced by the same cells, it is possible to theorize that the production of this hormone would also be inhibited. It has been reported that patients with adrenal failure and high ACTH production have a greatly increased incidence of hyperthyroidism.

TESTS OF THYROID FUNCTION

From the foregoing discussion of the effects of the thyroid hormone, it is apparent that many tests could be devised to measure its activity. The present battery includes several with reasonable reliabilities: These tests are given here not as a clinical problem but to illustrate the effect of the thyroid on metabolic processes and the factors influencing these processes.

1. *BMR.* One of the oldest tests, and the only one permitting direct quantitation of the animal's overall energy metabolism, is the determination of the basal metabolic rate (BMR). This test measures oxygen consumption under postabsorptive conditions and compares the results obtained to those of normal individuals. Results in human beings are reported as percentage increase or decrease from the normal reference value.

2. *PBI.* It has been previously mentioned that when the proteins of plasma are precipitated with suitable agents, T_4 and T_3 present are completely carried down. By analyzing the precipitate for iodine, the amount of thyroid hormone can be estimated. This is relatively constant in the normal person and usually varies from 4 to 8 milligrams per 100 milliliters of plasma. In hypothyroidism, the values fall below this and range about 1.5 milligrams per 100 milliliters.

In most instances, the PBI (protein-bound iodine) furnishes a clear indication of thyroid hormone output, but it remains an inadequate analysis of dynamic relationships between output and utilization (plus excretion) of hormone. Determination of radioactivity in the PBI (PBI^{131}) after administration of radioactive iodide (I^{131}) or (I^{125}) can furnish information about turnover of thyroxine.

3. *Radioactive iodine uptake.* The amount of iodine taken into the thyroid of an individual is a function of thyroid activity involving the rate of synthesis and the rate of release of thyroid hormone. Net thyroid activity can be estimated by giving minute doses of I^{131}, and measuring the amount of activity present in the thyroid after a definite time interval. The actual method is very simple since the patient is required only to drink a small amount of water containing the isotope and to sit in front of a Geiger-Muller or scintillation counter for a few minutes while the radioactive iodine in the neck region is estimated.

From the viewpoint of the biophysicist, the problem is not so simple. Radioactive iodines have a biological, as well as a physical, half-life. The latter is a constant; the time in which half the activity disappears. The former is the time required for half of the material to disappear from the body, or from a given organ; this varies from organ to organ and cannot adequately be taken into consideration. The problem is complicated further by the dilution of the minute amount of radioactive material administered with a large amount of nonradioactive iodine already present in the metabolic pool of the body. The assumption must be made that the radioactive iodine is distributed with and follows the exact pathways of the nonradioactive material. Finally, processes within the thyroid itself complicate the interpretation. Although the test may be called "uptake," it is again a measurement of the status of uptake versus release, both processes proceeding simultaneously.

Usually, a single determination is made in the human being at 24 hours. At that time, the typical hypothyroid patient will have less than 10 percent of the administered I^{131} in the thyroid; the euthyroid individual, from 20 to 40 percent; and the thyrotoxic patient, 60 percent or greater. For a more complete analysis, it is better to have values at two times, such as 4 hours and 24 hours. When an individual has had an uptake study, it is subsequently possible to follow the release of thyroid hormone. It is necessary to block reincorporation of I^{131} by administration of thiouracil; then, the rate of loss of radioactivity from the thyroid is measured. Injection of T_3 or T_4 will block, and TSH will enhance, the release rate. Release rate is generally interpreted in terms of endogenous TSH activity. Exogenous TSH can obviously be assayed by this procedure.

4. *Other methods.* Other methods of determining thyroid function are far less specific. There is a marked rise in serum cholesterol in the hypothyroid person, inversely related to the metabolic activity. Although cholesterol levels are lowered in hyperthyroidism, such changes are far less consistent. There is a tendency toward creatinuria in thyrotoxicosis; a creatine-tolerance test was once used, but it was abandoned in favor of the more specific functional tests discussed.

5. *T_4 and T_3.* Chromatographic and mass spectrometer assays now permit assays of T_3 and T_4 directly. Assays of the free hormone are obviously of great value in cases of protein disturbance. The techniques are troublesome because of the small amounts of hormone, but in capable hands they can render valuable information.

References

Tepperman, J. *The Thyroid in Metabolic and Endocrine Physiology*, 3rd ed. New York: Yearbook Publishing, 1974.
Inbar, S. H. and K. A. Woeber. *The thyroid gland.* In *Textbook of Endocrinology.* Edited by R. H. Williams. 5th ed. Baltimore: Williams & Wilkins, 1974.
Greep, R. D. and E. B. Astwood. *The Thyroid.* The Handbook of Physiology, sec. 7 vol. III. Washington, D.C.: American Physiology Society, 1974. Complete with thousands of references.

7
The Adrenal Gland

The small size of the adrenal gland in the adult (10 grams in the male, slightly larger in the female) belies the wide variety of activity carried out by this essential organ. The adrenal secretes steroid hormones important in the regulation of protein, fat, carbohydrate metabolism, and salt and water balance, and is essential to life. It is also an important member of the sympathetic nervous system.

If the adrenal gland is cut in cross section, two distinct layers can be seen (Figure 7.1). There is an inner, darkly pigmented center section, the *medulla*, which is completely surrounded by the lighter, yellowish cortex. The two areas comprise two different glands with no functional interrelationship despite their close proximity.

The two parts of the gland have a common blood supply. Blood from several adrenal arteries arising from the aorta, the renal, or other nearby arteries enters the cortex, breaks into sinusoids, and drains through the cortex to the medulla, after which it is collected into a single adrenal vein. This type of blood supply has advantages from the experimental viewpoint, since it is possible to cannulate the vein and obtain the total hormone production. At one time, it was believed that this type of drainage was required so that the hormone or hormone precursors produced by the cortex could be activated by passing through the medulla, but this view is no longer tenable. It is possible to separate the medulla and the cortex in the convoluted adrenal gland and shell out the medulla, leaving the cortex only partly damaged. In animals treated in this manner, the normal secre-

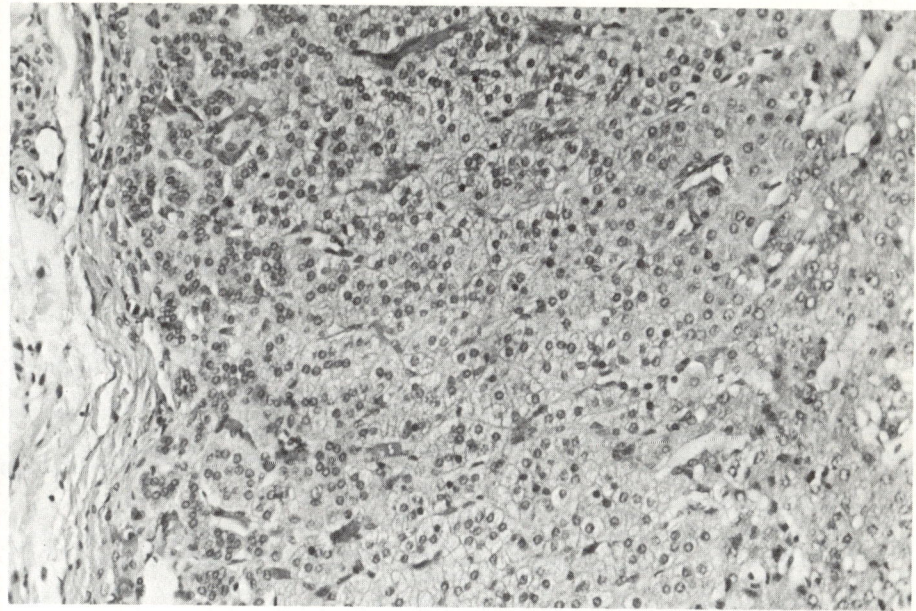

Figure 7.1. A microphotograph of the adrenal cortex showing the three major layers of the cortex.

tion of the cortex continues, demonstrating the independence of one gland from the other.

In addition, the secretions of the medulla and the cortex are chemically quite different. The cortex secretes a variety of steroid hormones, whereas the medulla secretes two catecholamine autonomic mediators, epinephrine and norepinephrine. The glands differ in another way. Denervation stops the function of the medulla, since it is essentially a ganglion of the autonomic nervous system; regeneration of secreting medullary cells is minimal. The cortex, on the other hand, is not altered by denervation and regenerates easily. If a relatively small number of cortical cells remain after removal of the larger part of the gland, the entire adrenal cortex can be restored with complete return of both structure and function.

THE ADRENAL CORTEX

If a cross section of the adrenal cortex is examined under the microscope, three distinct layers can be seen. There is an outer zone consisting of cells arranged in whorls or loops, the *zona glomerulosa;* a middle zone consisting of long cords of cells running toward the center of the gland, the *zona fasciculata;* and an innermost layer consisting of cells arranged in masses with no distinct order, the *zona reticularis.* The areas are marked off to some extent by connective tissue fibers, and the cellular arrangement is supported by connective tissue.

In addition to the three zones already mentioned, the human infant has a fourth layer of the gland, which lies next to the medulla and is called the *fetal X-zone.*

Control of the Adrenal Cortex. The size of the adrenal cortex and its rate of secretion are controlled by the anterior pituitary under the specific regulation of ACTH. Recall that ACTH is in turn controlled by CRF and possibly CIF (corticotrophic inhibiting factor) from the hypothalamus. If the pituitary is removed (hypophysectomy) or destroyed, the adrenal cortex decreases in size and in secretory ability. The gland shrinks to about 40 percent of the original weight, the loss being confined solely to the two inner zones. There is an apparent thickening of the zona glomerulosa, but this seems due to a rearrangement of cells as the cortex shrinks, rather than to an increase in number of size of cells in this layer. The glomerulosa secretes the steroids responsible for maintenance of salt and water balance; thus, the hypophysectomized animal does not die as does the completely adrenalectomized animal.

If one adrenal is removed, the output of ACTH increases and the remaining adrenal hypertrophies until it can assume the original output of both glands. On the other hand, if exogenous adrenocortical steroids are administered to an animal, the production of ACTH by the pituitary decreases, and the adrenal gland shrinks to the size of that in the hypophysectomized animal. Administration of exogenous ACTH will result in increased size and steroid output by the adrenal.

These observations lead to the usual feedback theory of adrenal control. ACTH from the pituitary causes growth of the adrenals and secretion into the bloodstream of steroids, some of which reach the pituitary and cause a decrease in the output of ACTH. Inhibition of ACTH production by implantation of a cortisone crystal in the pituitary is one piece of evidence supporting a direct feedback

THE ADRENAL GLAND   113

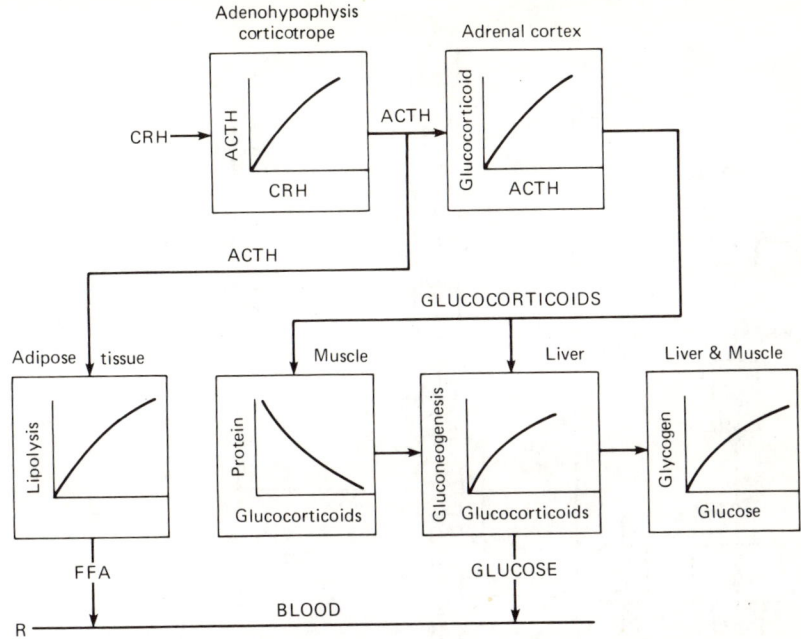

Figure 7.2. The control of the glucocorticoid secretion of the adrenal cortex indicating the widespread effects. (Taken from Kline, *Biological Foundations of Biomedical Engineering*, Little, Brown, Boston, 1976, with permission.)

mechanism. However, there is even more convincing support for hypothalamic participation in the feedback between the adrenal steroids and pituitary ACTH (see pp. 56–58), achieved through CRF.

The highly simplified control diagram in Figure 7.2 illustrates the major site of action of the adrenal steroids. The liver, the muscle, and adipose tissue further suggest the action on protein and carbohydrate metabolism. On the other hand, Figure 7.3 indicates the major control points including blood volume, atrial receptors, the kidney-renin system, and the other inputs including ADH that help to control cortisol secretion. Note also that Figure 7.3 includes the effect of protein-binding of cortisol on its activity. The reader can easily supply the curves at each point showing the system response.

Considerable evidence suggests that ACTH has its major stimulatory effect on the two inner zones of the adrenal cortex, exerting a relatively minor, but by no means negligible, effect on the zona

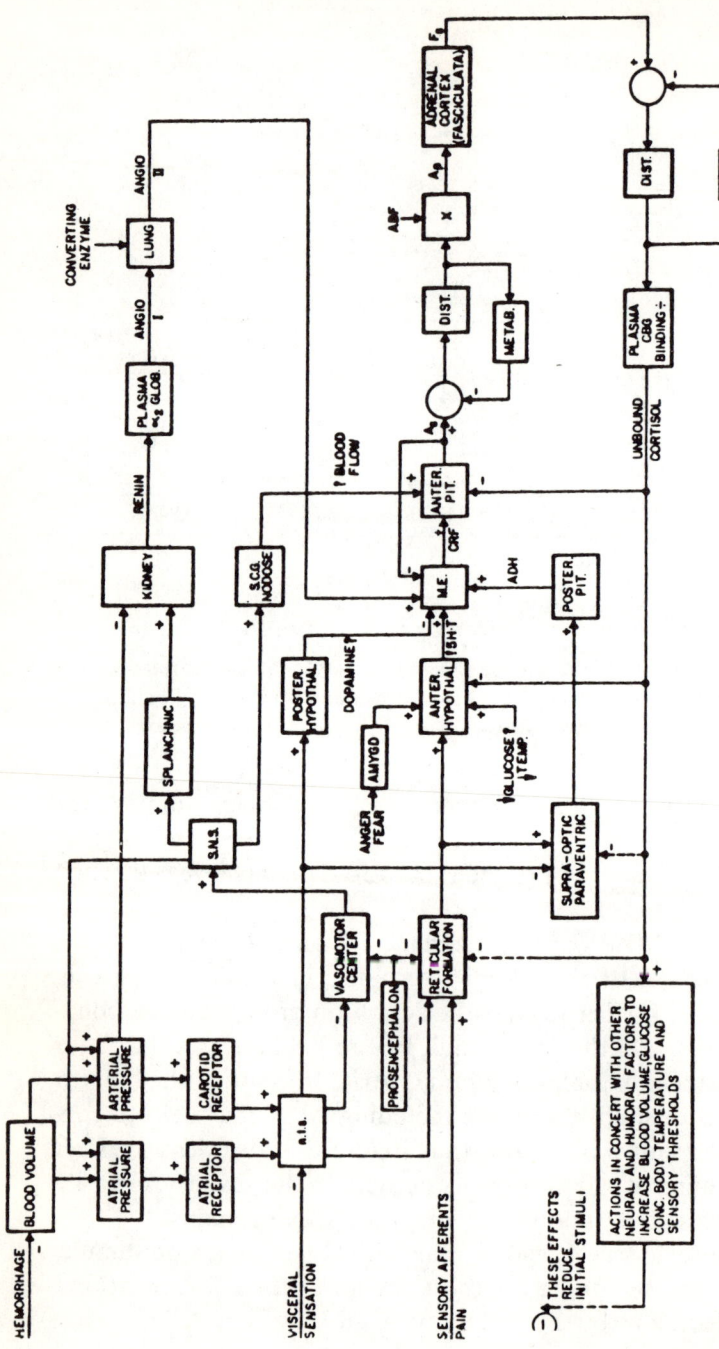

Figure 7.3. Diagram of overall system controlling secretion of cortisol. Note the multiple parallel paths. Symbols: +, increase or stimula; −, decrease of irhibition; A_s, adrenocorticotropin secreted; A_p, adrenocorticotrophin presented; ABF, adrenal blood flow; F_s, cortisol d; dist., distribution; metab., metabolism; CBG, cortisol-binding globulin; angio, angiotensin; CRF, corticotrophin-releasing factor; superior cervical ganglion; n.t.s., nucleus tractus solitarius; M.E., median eminence; 5H-T, 5-hydroxytryptamine; ADH, vasopressin. (Taken from Brown and Gann, *Engineering Principles in Physiology*, Academic Press, New York, 1975, with permission.)

glomerulosa and production of the electrocorticoid hormone *aldosterone*, which is controlled through an entirely separate process.

The control system that regulates the secretion of aldosterone is diagramed in Figure 7.4. The exact triggering mechanism is not known, but apparently decreased body-fluid volume, blood volume, or pressure in some way stimulates the production of renin by the kidney. Renin is a protease that converts a glycoprotein in alpha globulin of plasma to angiotensin I by cleaving the molecule, and then angiotensin II is formed from angiotensin I by enzymes in the blood, which are stimulated by the pituitary and adrenocortical hormones. Angiotensin II is then able to stimulate the production of aldosterone by the glomerulosa of the adrenal. Aldosterone then stimulates the kidney tubule to retain sodium, and as a consequence, water. Low sodium or high potassium concentration also affects the system by stimulating the glomerulosa directly, and ADH operates by stimulating the tubule directly. The end result is the overall effect of all the factors working together. Regulation of aldosterone secretion is known to depend upon levels of sodium, potassium, and extracellular fluid volume operating through kidney secretion of renin. Studies by Davis et al. and Ganong et al. have clearly demonstrated some involvement of the renin-angiotensin humoral pathway in stimulating aldosterone secretion. There is no question, however, that both the anterior pituitary and hypothalamus will, when stimulated, increase the production of aldosterone. The exact relationships between renin mechanisms and other means

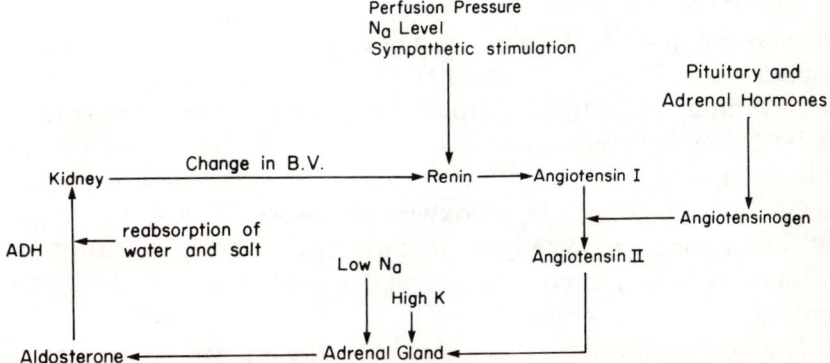

Figure 7.4. The control system for the secretion of aldosterone. Note the difference in control from Figure 7.2 for the glucocorticoids.

of stimulation are not clear. It is also apparent that the renin system stimulates ADH production with resultant effects on water balance.

The Adrenal Steroids. The adrenal cortex elaborates hormones that fall into the general classification of steroids. The name is derived from cholesterine, coined by Michel Chevreul for material isolated from bile. Some understanding of the chemistry of the molecule is necessary in order to relate to structure to function, not only in hormones of the adrenal cortex but also in the estrogens and androgens, which are also steroids.

The basic steroid molecule consists of four carbon rings fused together. Three rings (A, B, C) are six-membered rings, while the fourth (D) is five-membered (Figure 7.5). Seventeen carbon atoms are involved, with specific numbers as shown. In addition, there are usually two other carbon atoms (numbered 18 and 19) attached as methyl groups to the thirteenth and tenth carbon atoms of the ring system, respectively; these are usually indicated only by the bond marks. In the adrenocortical steroids (but not necessarily in other steroids), there is a side chain of two carbon atoms (20 and 21) attached to the seventeenth carbon of the ring system. In the "parent" compound, the rings are completely saturated (the pregnane nucleus), and by convention the hydrogens are not usually indicated.

A closer study reveals that the ring system contains eight asymmetric carbon atoms with 256 possible steroisomers. Actually, only a few of these are known, and fewer still are of biological importance.

The major corticosteroids secreted by adrenals of adult male humans are given in Figure 7.5, together with chemical and trivial names. It will be noticed that they bear certain characteristic substitutions. All adrenal steroids have a ketone group on carbon-3 and a double bond between carbons-4 and -5. Each has a two-carbon side-chain with a ketone on carbon-20 and an alcohol grouping on carbon-21. There may be an oxygen on carbon-11, and, in the case of aldosterone, an aldehyde at carbon-18. These substitutions produce certain definite changes in the biological activity of the molecule.

The present evidence indicates that the human adrenal gland secretes a mixture of the aforementioned steroids with about 85 percent of the output consisting of cortisol. Corticosterone and

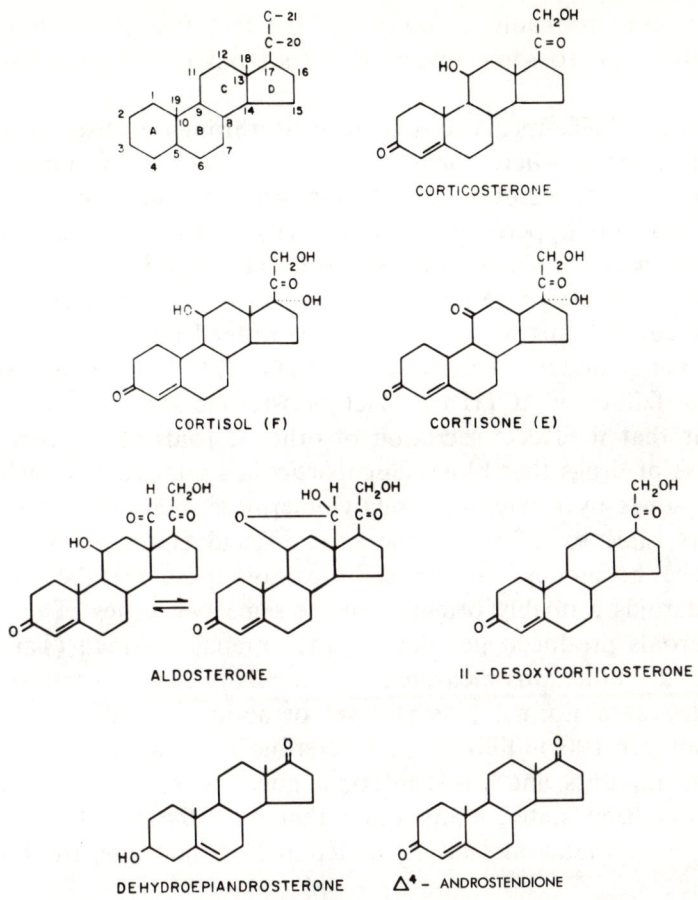

Figure 7.5. The steroid nucleus indicating the numbering of the carbon atoms and some commonly occurring adrenal steroids—corticosterone as a parent compound; cortisol and cortisone as glucocorticoids; aldosterone and 11-desoxycorticosterone as electrocorticoids; and dehydroepiandrosterone and androstenedione as androgens. Progesterone and estradiol are also present in small quantities.

aldosterone are the most important of the remaining corticosteroids secreted. In addition to those already mentioned, examination of the blood and urine reveals several other steroids. It is not always certain how many of these are degradation products of tissue metabolism, how many are precursors of adrenal steroid synthesis, and how many are products of the analytical method. The close relationship of structure probably accounts for the fact that most steroids apparently bind to some extent to all steroid receptors in the target cells.

The feedback regulation is probably through cortisol because, in certain diseases where cortisol is not produced (as the adrenogenital syndrome), the secretion of ACTH is extremely high, and the adrenal gland remains hyperactive despite a large output of other steroids. The feedback for aldosterone will be discussed later.

There appears to be a relationship between structure and function in the adrenal cortex. It has been mentioned that the zona glomerulosa is not under the direct control of ACTH. This is substantiated by the failure of ACTH to affect aldosterone secretion to the same extent that it effects secretion of other steroids of the cortex. By the use of drugs that block glucocorticoid synthesis and destroy the inner zones by leaving the zona glomerulosa intact (amphenone B), it is possible to infer that the zona fasciculata and zona reticularis produce hormones concerned in carbohydrate metabolism. The ketosteroids probably originate in the same two zones. The amount of steroids produced per day by the adrenals is small (Table 7.1). About 25 milligrams measured as cortisol are excreted into the urine per day at a normal plasma level of about 25 milligrams of free cortisol per 100 milliliters. Aldosterone is produced in even more minute amounts, and less than 100 nanograms are excreted per day.

It has been stated many times that only the *free* hormone can perform its metabolic duties; under most conditions, the hormone

Table 7.1. Adrenal steroid secretion in normal adult males.*

Group	Compound	Mean 24-Hour Secretion
Glucocorticoids	Cortisol	15–30 mg
	Corticosterone	2–5 mg
Mineralocorticoids	Aldosterone	50–150 µg
	11-Desoxycorticosterone	Trace
Androgens	Dehydroepiandrosterone	15–30 mg
	-Androstenedione	0–10 mg
	11-Hydroxyandrostenedione	0–10 mg
Proestins	Progesterone	0.4–0.8 mg
Estrogens	Estradiol	Trace

*Data assembled by Dr. R. E. Taylor, Jr.

circulating in the bloodstream is bound or complexed to some component, usually protein, in the plasma. This is also true of the adrenal steroids. Cortisol is bound to two proteins when it enters the bloodstream. Transcortin, which is a globulin, has an extremely high affinity for cortisol but a relatively low capacity. Albumin, on the other hand, has a low affinity but an almost unlimited binding capacity. (The relationship of changing binding capacity to free hormone has been discussed in the section on the thyroid, p. 96.) In pregnancy, high estrogen levels cause an increase in the globulin or transcortin in the plasma, and the binding of cortisol rises from 75 to about 95 percent; thus, the determination of cortisol in pregnancy usually shows levels higher than normal but with increased binding. The amount of *active* steroid may not be significantly increased.

The steroids produced by the adrenals are secreted into the bloodstream and carried to the tissues where they perform their functions. In various tissues, but primarily the liver, the steroids are changed to less active forms or to conjugated forms and then excreted by the kidney. As a result, the blood always contains active steroid on the way to the liver and other tissues, and inactive forms on the way to excretion by the kidney from the site of inactivation.

One step in the process of elimination of steroids via the urine involves conjugation of the water-insoluble molecule with a material that makes it more water-soluble, such as glucuronic acid or sulfuric acid. As a result of the conjugation, the blood and urine contain both free and esterified steroids, with the concentration of the latter several times that of the former.

The synthesis of the adrenocorticol steroids is illustrated in Figure 7.6. This figure explains the clinical syndromes that are characterized by failure of the synthetic mechanism at one point or another. ACTH appears to act at a point preceding the formation of pregnenolone. The androgens that are formed by the adrenal cortex are probably derived after the formation of pregnenolone, since their output is usually increased by ACTH.

Metabolic Paths. Figure 7.6 illustrates the main pathways of steroid metabolism in the adrenal cortex. It also shows the effects of metabolic disease, which occurs through the block of particular enzymes or the genetic absence of enzymes. If the enzyme that serves to convert the β-ol to the aldehyde is missing, all of the

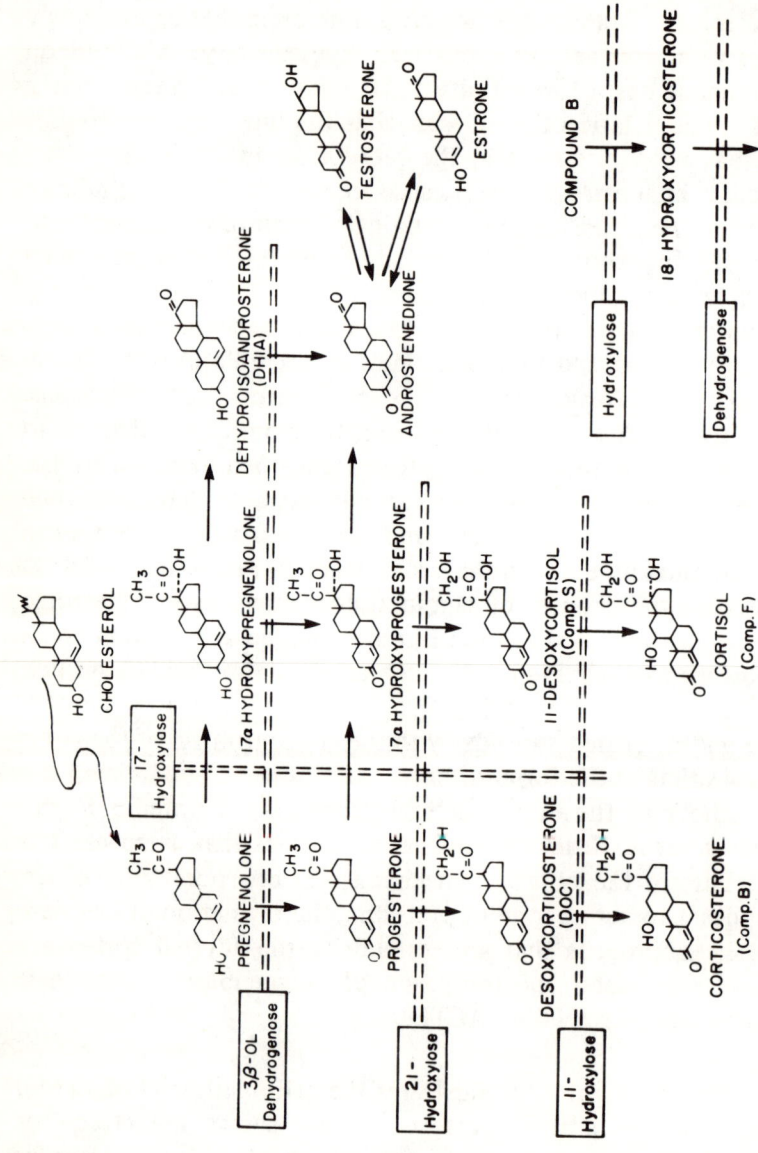

Figure 7.6. The metabolic pathways for the synthesis of the adrenocortical steroids, indicating the major enzymatic reactions.

products are diverted into the androgen pathways. Masculinization is to be expected. On the other hand, the absence of a carbon-21 hydrolase prevents the conversion of progesterones to adrenal steroids, and the absence of 11-hydrolase prevents the formation of the carbohydrate-regulating steroids and cortisol, which is the feedback to the pituitary. In this case, large amounts of desoxycorticosterone, which is a potent salt-retaining steroid, are produced. In each case, the basic phenomenon is the same. The steroid serving as the feedback for ACTH production is not produced, so more ACTH is excreted and the adrenal is stimulated to produce more abnormal steroids. Each of the diseases responds to the same treatment as could be expected from the knowledge of the control system. Adminstration of cortisol returns ACTH and adrenal secretion to normal but, of course, does not correct the metabolic defect.

The steroids of adrenal origin that appear in the blood consist mainly of the corticoids (cortisol, cortiosterone, aldosterone) and the androgens (androstenedione, 11-hydroxyandrostenedione, dehydroisoandrosterone). In the process of metabolism, these compounds are converted to other, less active structures. In general, adrenal corticoids are reduced to the *tetrahydro-* forms of the original steroid, and those with a 17-hyroxyl may also be converted to 17-ketosteroids, both processes occurring predominantly in the liver. Those without a 17-hydroxy group do not produce 17-ketosteroids and are excreted in conjugated forms.

It should be emphasized that any diagram of relationship among steroids is highly tentative, especially when the evidence is based on urinary excretory products. All of the steroids that are present in blood, whether degradation products or freshly formed steroids from the adrenal, are excreted in the urine. The only sure method for determining metabolites from the natural products is to examine urine and gland steroid output stimultaneously. By quantitating the output of the gland following cannulations of the adrenal vein, especially under ACTH stimulation, it is possible to determine which of the steroids are synthesized there. The additional steroids found in the urine must be metabolic products formed in the peripheral tissues.

Many major difficulties beset the individual following the pathways of steroid metabolism. One of the most difficult problems has been the failure to find completely satisfactory methods for the extraction, analysis, and recovery of administered steroids. Less than 50 percent of an administered dose of steroid can be recovered in all possible known forms as the result of inadequate techniques plus total destruction of much of the material.

Physical methods have been devised within the past few years, which greatly improve the chances of identification of a specific steroid. Many of the steroids fluoresce at specific wavelengths determined by the structure of the molecule, and this can be used for identification. The infrared spectrum of each steroid is highly specific for its structure. However, both of these methods depend to a large extent on a high degree of purity of the compound tested. Fortunately, the development of column and paper chromatography has greatly aided the steroid chemist in the resolution of mixtures of steroids, and thus in identification. The recent improvements in the mass spectrometer make it possible to determine femtogram (10^{-13}) quantities of steroids and to determine the structure and molecular weight accurately and quickly. When combined with a gas chromatograph to separate various compounds and with computer control to enhance accuracy and speed, the mass spectrometer has become the invaluable tool of the steroid chemist.

A more serious problem is presented in biological assay of the steroids. Vast numbers of tests have been proposed as assays, each based upon a biological property of adrenocortical steroids in living tissue. The inherent difficulties appear insurmountable. Any one test appears to be reasonably reproducible, and a certain pattern emerges for all tests taken together, but there is no agreement as to the potency of a preparation as determined by several tests. This again may reflect problems in competitive binding at receptor sites.

Despite the difficulties of assessing test results, generalizations can be made. It is apparent that compounds that have an oxygen at the 11-position are active in those assays involving a test of carbohydrate metabolism. The compounds with no oxygen at the 11-position are, in general, active in those tests involving salt metabolism and maintenance of life. Aldosterone is an outstanding exception since it does have an 11-hydroxy; however, this can exist in a tautomeric ring form including the 18-keto group, a situation that strongly alters the activity. In those compounds on which a 17-hydroxy has been placed, enhancement of activity on carbohydrate metabolism is apparent over the parent compound. Recent efforts of steroid

Table 7.2. Assay of naturally occurring steroids by various methods.

In each case, a specific steroid has been taken as a reference and assigned a value of 100, and the other steroids are compared to it in terms of percent activity.

Steroid	Survival After Adrenalectomy	Sodium Retention	Ingle's Work Test	Effect on Carbohydrate Metabolism	Ability to Withstand Stress (Cold)	Liver Glycogen Deposition
Desoxycorticosterone	100	100	1	25	10	1
Cortisol	55	5	100	100	100	100
Corticosterone	70	15	34	70	9	33
Reichstein's S	10	1	1	25	2	0
Aldosterone	2,000	2,500	10		80	21

A comparison of the activity of the newer synthetic steroids in terms of hydrocortisone.

Compound	Common Name*	Glycogen Deposition	Na Retention DOC = 100	Anti-Inflammatory	Survival
Hydrocortisone	Cortisol	100	5	100	100
9-Fluorohydrocortisone	Fluorocortisone	800	500	600	4
Δ^1-6-CH$_3$-Hydrocortisone	Mehtylprednisolone	1,000	**	600	—
Δ^1-Hydrocortisone	Prednisolone	300	**	300	200
Δ^1-16-OH-9-Fluorohydrocortisone	Triamcinolone	3,350	**	650	—
Δ^1-16-CH$_3$-9-Fluorohydrocortisone	Dexamethasone	1,500	**	2,000	—

*A variety of registered names exists for each of these compounds.
**Sodium and water retention caused by these materials is usually stated to be very low or absent. In the case of human patients, the prolonged treatment often required sometimes does produce serious edema.

chemists have involved the alteration of the molecule in such a way as to increase a desired activity (Table 7.2). For example, the inclusion of a fluorine bond at position 1, greatly increases the activity affecting carbohydrate metabolism. The mechanism by which any specific structure affects a particular activity is unknown.

METABOLIC EFFECTS OF ADRENOCORTICAL HORMONES

Administration of the adrenal hormones, particularly those of the 17-hydroxy type, results in a rise in blood sugar, which may persist for some time when the steroids are withdrawn. This elevation in blood sugar has been called *steroid diabetes* and occurs because of a combination of accelerated gluconeogenesis plus depressed carbohydrate oxidation. Since proteins are the principal source of the blood sugar, there is accelerated proteolysis, the resulting amino acids are deaminated, and the carbon skeletons of the molecules are delivered into the metabolic pool to be broken down and resynthesized into glucose.

The diabetes produced by steroids is not due to the failure of glucose to enter the cells as in pancreatic diabetes. Therefore insulin has very little effect on the course of the blood sugar, and the experimental diabetes is called *insulin resistant*. The amount of nitrogen or protein catabolism cannot account for the entire rise in blood sugar, and it is concluded that the adrenal hormones also exert an inhibitory effect on the utilization of glucose in the periphery. Experiments in the highly insulin-sensitive hypophysectomized dog indicate that cortisone administration decreases but does not entirely abolish the insulin hypersensitivity, suggesting that some additional factor is involved in the normal *antiinsulin effect* of the pituitary. This factor may be the pituitary growth hormone or some other unidentified *diabetogenic* principle.

In the adrenalectomized animal, peripheral utilization of glucose is enhanced, and the formation of glucose from protein is impeded. As a result of the inability to carry out gluconeogenesis, the animal becomes insulin-sensitive and, on fasting, readily develops hypoglycemia. This explains the report of Long and Lukens that adrenalectomy ameliorates diabetes by lowering blood sugar and improving the utilization of glucose. It is also partially the basis for the similar decrease in the severity of diabetes observed by Houssay after hypophysectomy.

The negative nitrogen balance following stress may be explained by the same sequence. During any type of stress to the individual, the adrenal cortex is activated via the hypothalamic pathway, and the output of steroid increases. This in turn increases the blood sugar through gluconeogensis and increases nitrogen excretion from protein catabolism. This effect does not occur in the adrenalectomized animal but will take place in such an animal given maintenance doses of cortisone. This is an example of "permissive" action of the adrenal, where a small amount of steroid is required to support a metabolic process, which then is able to respond to other controls.

From the effects of the adrenal on carbohydrate metabolism, it is not difficult to explain its effect on protein metabolism. The increased excretion of nitrogen, primarily as urea, as a result of gluconeogenesis caused by the adrenal steroids has already been mentioned. That this process continues in the eviscerated animal supports the contention of some researchers that major catabolism of protein under the influence of corticoids occurs in the peripheral tissues without the necessary participation of the liver. Furthermore, experiments measuring nitrogen metabolism by turnover of N^{15} demonstrate that the adrenal not only increases catabolism of protein but that it also inhibits protein anabolism, depending upon the size of the metabolic pool upon which the animal can draw. It is also possible that many other factors, such as alteration in salt balance and blood volume, in the adrenalectomized animal could produce aberrant results that are not directly a metabolic defect. There is some evidence that increased steroid levels promote synthesis of protein in the liver, even in the presence of an overall negative nitrogen balance. This suggest that the liver may respond to steroids in a different manner than the peripheral tissues.

Because of the close interrelationship of carbohydrate, fat, and protein metabolism, it would be suprising if the adrenal cortex did not have an effect on lipogenesis. There is some evidence that adrenalectomy increases fat formation in the animal on a high carbohydrate diet. If this loss of control over lipogenesis occurs during fasting, it may contribute to the hypoglycemia and depletion of liver glycogen regularly observed in the adrenalectomized animal. If animals are partially depancreatized to produce a mild diabetes and are then given cortisone, the ketonuria and the severity of the diabetes are increased. Although these results would seem to indicate that the adrenal hormones increase oxidation of fat, large doses

126   INTEGRATION AND COORDINATION OF METABOLIC PROCESSES

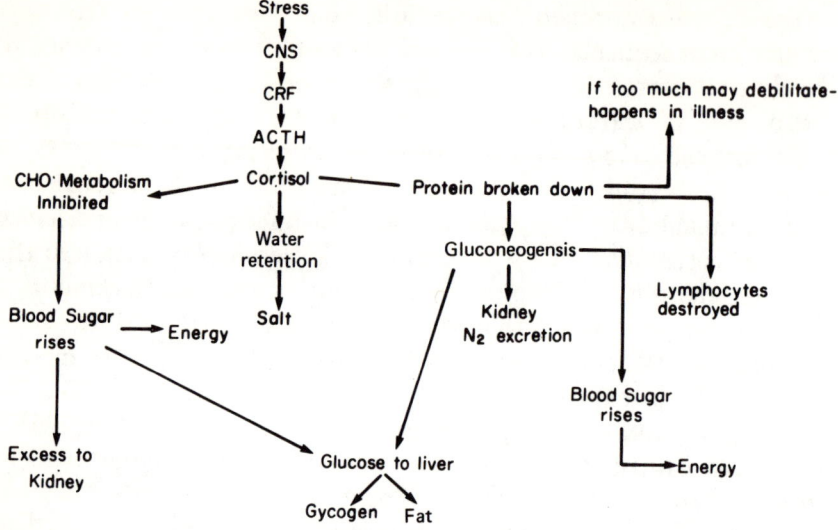

Figure 7.7. The major effects of the glucocorticoids on carbohydrate, fat, and protein metabolism.

of cortisone have been shown to increase fat deposition, and, in some forms of adrenal hypersecretion, fatty deposits occur, although these are not distributed normally.

The complex interrelationship between protein, carbohydrate, water, and fat metabolism under the influence of the glucocorticoids is shown in Figure 7.7. The breakdown of protein, water retention, inhibition of carbohydrate metabolism, and the increase in fat deposition are clearly shown to be interrelated. It must be remembered, however, that small amounts of the glucocorticoids are necessary to provide "permissive" action before many of the anabolic processes can proceed. Further interrelationship between the adrenal cortex and other hormones in the control of the same processes are shown in Figure 7.7. Recall the relationship of GH, TSH, insulin, and ACTH to the control of metabolism and the effect of the adrenal, posterior pituitary, and parathyroid on water and salt excretion.

Salt and Water Metabolism. The adrenal cortex has a profound effect on salt metabolism, largely through the activity of the mineralocorticoid, aldosterone. In the absence of the cortex, the excretion of sodium increases, the plasma sodium level drops materially, and plasma potassium rises. The excretion of water parallels that of sodium probably as an osmotic phenomenon. The effect appears to reside largely in the failure of the ability of the kidney tubules to reabsorb sodium and to excrete potassium due to the lack of aldosterone. The increased absorption of potassium that accompanies the increased sodium excretion following adrenalectomy is probably an obligatory process, in which the kidney returns to the blood the univalent potassium ion for the univalent sodium ion that the tubules can no longer reabsorb effectively. The loss of sodium alters the osmotic balance between extracellular and intracellular compartments, and water passes into the cells. This results in hemoconcentration, fall in blood pressure, and bradycardia. The changes can be reversed in the adrenalectomized rat and in some human hypoadrenal cases by oral replacement of the salt loss. In order to avoid cardiac depression from the high serum potassium, the level of this salt in the diet must be greatly restricted. It should be emphasized that salt replacement does not completely restore the animal to normal and that many other dangers to life exist in adrenocortical insufficiency.

In the absence of the adrenocortical steroids (largely aldosterone), there is a marked water retention under water-loading; the animal deprived of these steroids appears unable to excrete water in the normal fashion. A large portion of this defect must be due to the loss of salt, the changing osmotic relations of the plasma, and the entrance of water into the cells. The low blood pressure lowers the glomerular filtration rate and renal plasma flow, and this contributes to the failure of water excretion. There is also some evidence that ADH secretion is triggered by a deficiency of adrenal steroids, which could lead to water retention. It should be remembered that overdosage of an animal with certain adrenal steroids will also cause water retention, largely because of the increased reabsorption of sodium and the water that must go with it to maintain osmotic equilibrium. However, this is not the entire picture, because prolonged administration of desoxycorticosterone (DOC), for example, will result in a sort of diabetes insipidus in which there is a high water intake and output with very low salt excretion. There is also some evidence of alteration of permeability of the cells to ions in the presence of adrenal steroids.

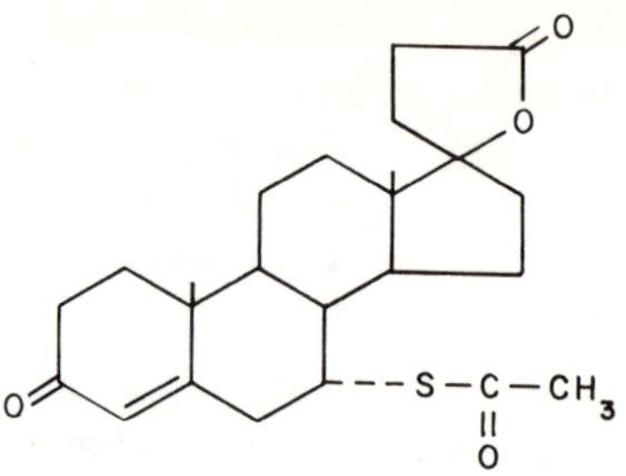

Figure 7.8. The structure of spirolactone (Aldactone A), a structural antagonistic of aldosterone. Note the similarity to the steroids.

Aldosterone acts by entering the cytosol of the kidney cells where it is bound to receptors. Very little aldosterone enters the nucleus of the cells. There is some evidence that steroid hormones, which must produce their effects on DNA by entering the nucleus (estrogens and progesterone), require a long-term binding in order to produce an effect, while those steroids such as aldosterone, which affect cell permeability, may not require nuclear activity and require only short-term contact with the cell. The compound spiralactone (Figure 7.8), which blocks the actions of aldosterone, does not compete for the same sites but operates at another part of the RNA stimulation path.

Various portions of the central nervous system, including the hypothalamus, pituitary, and even the pineal body, have been implicated in the entire adrenoglomerulotrophin picture, with suggestions that some communicating structures are themselves sensitive to changes in pulse pressure, vascular distention, or electrolyte concentration. Potential relationships are shown in Figure 7.3, including the possibility that ACTH itself may play a small role, either as a permissive agent to establish adrenocortical responsiveness, or as a direct but low-level glomerulosa-stimulating factor.

Aldosterone injection can rectify the defects in salt metabolism seen in the adrenalectomized animal, but it seems to be unable to correct water retention, and it does not produce the *diabetes insipidus effect* of DOC. It may still be too early to dismiss a possible physiological role for DOC.

Other Effects of Adrenalectomy. Many of the defects produced by adrenalectomy cannot be attributed to the metabolic functions of the gland. They are extremely diverse in character, and no common traits are found among them. These include:

1. *Asthenia and Fatigue of Muscle.* This is characteristic of adrenalectomized individuals and is so reproducible that methods of assay of adrenal steroids have been based on the phenomenon, such as the muscle work test of Dwight Ingle. It is not yet certain whether this is a true defect of the contractile mechanism produced by the absence of adrenal steroids or if it is due to defects in cell metabolism, blood flow, and so on, which occur following adrenalectomy. In general, the defect is relieved by the glucocorticoids rather than electrocorticoids.

2. *Cardiovascular System.* In addition to the effects of adrenalectomy on the cardiovascular system, which may be explained on the basis of alteration in water or electrolyte balance, there are characteristic changes in capillary function. An increased permeability develops, which may be due to alterations in integrity of the capillary wall, to diminished vascular tone and vasoconstriction, or to other unknown factors. The responsiveness of the system to sympathetic stimulation appears to diminish more than would be expected as a result of loss of medullary tissue. This leads to inability of the system to compensate for stress by shunting blood to stressed areas and tends to make the adrenalectomized animal more sensitive to such factors.

3. *Lymphatic System.* In the absence of the adrenal, a generalized hyperplasia of the lymphatic system occurs. This includes enlargement of the thymus, increase in the number of circulating lymphocytes, etc. Administration of steroids such as cortisone reverses this trend and causes regression of the thymus and decrease in circulating lymphocytes. Since the lymphocytes contain some of the basic antibody material, the *gamma globulins*, it has been suggested that the decrease in lymphocytes constitues a release of antibody and aids in the protection of the body against stress. There is little evidence that this is true. Other blood cells are similarly affected: the eosinophils decrease markedly when steroids are administered, and this has been widely used as a test of adrenal functions. The adrenalectomized animal usually has an anemia resulting from depression of the red bone marrow and failure of red-blood-cell synthesis.

4. *Connective Tissue.* The connective tissue is made up of three

major components: the fibroblast, the fiber itself, and ground substance. When tissue is damaged, the fibroblasts lay down new collagen fibers, and the ground substance is inhibited. Hyaluronic acid, another component of the ground substance, is broken down, probably by increased activity of the enzyme hyaluronidase, which facilitates spreading of many substances in tissues. The formation of new fibroblasts is inhibited. All of these processes result in delay in wound healing, formation of weak scars, and penetration of fibrin into the wound. In humans, one of the most serious of the collagen diseases is arthritis; the success of cortisone and similar compounds in its treatment may be due to inhibition of some of the mechanisms just outlined, with a resultant decrease in inflammation.

5. *Bone and Cartilage.* Increased secretion of adrenocortical hormones appears to decrease bone growth and to prevent proliferation of cartilage cells, and leads to osteoporosis and decalcification of the bone. This may be a result of excessive catabolism of protein in the bone as well as elsewhere in the body, with resulting failure to lay down the organic matrix into which minerals are deposited.

6. *Skin and Hair.* The growth of hair is suppressed, and the skin may become thinner. It is difficult to associate this directly with a deficiency of the known protein-mobilizing activity of the adrenal corticoids.

7. *Resistance to Stress.* The adrenalectomized animal is sensitive to a varity of applied stimuli ranging from trauma, cold, toxins, and durgs of many kinds, to circulatory shock, and possibly to other factors that are not understood. These agents stimulate the normal adrenal cortex to elaborate steroids, which in some way afford a protection that is lacking in the adrenal-deficient animal. The adrenal cortex is only one of a series of mechanisms involved in homeokinesis, the net dynamic regulation of physiological processes. The entire endocrine system is constantly in action as long as life exists, responding to weak as well as strong stimuli. It is probably as unfair to single out one endocrine gland as it is to consider the endocrine system specifically more important than the nervous system.

The reactions of the adrenal to stress must be mediated through the hypothalamus and the anterior pituitary, for hypophysectomized animals are also unable to respond to stress. Although epinephrine has been implicated as an agent that fires the pituitary to cause release of ACTH and stimulation of the cortex, present indications are that this constitues only a small, very prompt part of the total stimulation. This would suggest that two or more mechanisms are responsible for ACTH release, sympathetic stimulation, and other poorly defined factors in stress resistance.

The adrenal cortex has a close relationship with the other endocrine organs. The reciprocal balance between the cortex and the pancreas has already been discussed.

There is also a relationship between the adrenal steroids and the sex hormones in both male and female. The inner zones of the adrenal cortex are capable of producing androgens in relatively large quantity. The human female excretes in the urine about 6 to 10 milligrams of 17-ketosteroids per day, most of which probably originate from the adrenal. As already noted, andogenically active steroids are produced in the course of adrenocorticoid synthesis. In addition, the breakdown of adrenocortical steroids in the liver and elsewhere may yield 17-ketosteroids. There are certain metabolic diseases of the adrenal, such as the "adrenogenital syndrome," (p. 120) in which androgens are excreted in large amounts because of deficient activity of some enzymes concerned with synthesis of the adrenal corticoids. The relationship of the adrenal to the gonads is shown by data indicating that the suppression of FSH release by testosterone also results in decreased secretion of ACTH, thus producing smaller adrenal weight in test animals.

The larger adrenal:body-weight ratio in female rats than in males may be the result of some estrogen effect on adrenocortical function.

Relationship between the thyroid and the adrenal is apparent. Excess thyroid hormone administration constitutes a stress, with resultant adrenal hypertrophy probably due to the increased metabolic rate and the greater demands placed on the organism. There are some indications that thyroidectomy decreases the production of steroids by the adrenal and that adrenal corticoids in turn inhibit thyroid activity. The latter effect may be due to inadequate synthesis of thyroglobulin protein in the face of the protein catabolic activity of excess corticoids.

Assay of Corticoids. From the previous survey of the metabolic activities of the corticoids, methods of assay can be easily summarized. Assays have been proposed that measure glycogen deposition in liver, work rate of stimulated muscles, maintenance of life, diabetogenic activity, depletion of lymphoid tissue (eosinophil response), protection against various stresses, and retention or excretion of sodium and potassium. With a given steroid, the responses vary widely from test to test. Although chemical assay has become the method of choice, the student must never forget that ultimately all chemical assays must be related to a *biological* assay.

Hyperfunction of the adrenal cortex occurs in the adult, more often in the female than in the male, and involves a bilateral adrenal hyperplasia with overproduction of steroids. The excess steroid production results in accumulation of fat (largely on the face and back), osteoporosis, diabetes, salt retention, and hypertension, all of which can be predicted from Figure 7.7. In addition, excess production of androgens in the female causes virilism with baldness, development of a beard, and interference with normal menstrual cycles. This disease may be of either adrenal or pituitary origin. Differentiation can be made by administration of exogenous steroid to suppress the pituitary and decrease the output of the adrenal gland if the disease is not of "autonomous" origin.

Stress and the Adrenal Cortex. When an organism is exposed to a factor that threatens the normal homeokinetic balance, it is said to be stressed. The stressor that places the initial strain on the organism may be chemical, environmental, mental, or almost any other factor. In experimental work upon this phenomenon, the stresses most often applied have been those of heat, cold, traumatic injury, or similar processes that can be controlled in the laboratory. The organism must adapt itself to resist the stress when it is applied. The animal responds to the stress by releasing adrenocortical steroids, which, in a manner that is ill-understood, afford some protection against the applied force.

A general theory of reaction to stress, formulated by Hans Selye, is the *general adaption syndrome* (GAS), which involves three stages: (1) shock when the animal is initially exposed to the stress and must set up defenses to combat it, (2) resistance when the organism is able to adjust to the changed environment by the processes under the control of the adrenal cortex, and (3) exhaustion when the animal can no longer maintain its defenses against the encroaching stress. Selye has presented evidence to support this theory that many of the common diseases of the vascular system are the result of these processes. The theory has aroused great interest and much controversy, the latter primarily because of the overemphasis of pituitary-adrenal cortical predominance. Indeed, orthodoxy allows no role for other physiological systems. There appears to be a *stress phenomenon*, which does produce an outpouring of adrenocortical hormones, but it is by no means clear that it should be given the prominence outlined by Selye. It is also clear that many mechanisms other than the adrenal pituitary axis appear to be involved.

References

Christy, N. P. *The Human Adrenal Cortex*. New York: Harper & Row, 1971.
Fitzsimon, J. T. "Thirst." *Physiol. Rev.* 52 (1972): 468.
Freedman, M. A. and Freedman, S. N. *Introduction to Steroid Biochemistry and Its Clinical Allocation*. New York: Harper & Row, 1970.
Gill, G. "Mechanism of ACTH Action." *Metabolism* 21 (1972): 571.
Glaz, E. and P. Vecsei. *Aldosterone*. New York: Pergamon Press, 1971.
Laragh, J. H., L. Baer, A. R. Brunner, F. R. Buhler, J. E. Sealey, and E. D. Vaughan. "Renin Angiotensin and Aldosterone System in Pathogensis and Management of Hypertensive Vascular Disease." *Am. J. Med.* 52 (1972): 633.
Litwack, G., and S. Singer. "Subcellular Actions of Glucocorticoids." In G. Litwack (ed.), *Biochemical Actions of Hormones*. Vol. II. New York: Academic Press, 1972.
Muller, J. *Regulation of Aldosterone Biosynthesis*. New York: Springer-Verlag, 1971.
Mulrow, P. J. "The Adrenal Cortex." *Ann. Rev. Physiol.* 34 (1972): 409.
Sharp, G. W. G. and A. Leaf. "Mechanism of Action of Aldosterone." *Physiol. Rev.* 46 (1966): 593.
Stanbury, J. B., J. B. Wyngaarden, and D. S. Fredrickson. *The Metabolic Basis of Inherited Disease*. 3d ed. New York: McGraw-Hill, 1972.
Streeten, D. H. P. "The Spirolacton." *Clin. Pharmacol. & Therap.* 2 (1961): 359.

8
The Adrenal Medulla

The adrenal medulla is bivalent in its function in the body. The medulla is obviously of nervous origin, and its activity could lead one to classify it as a part of the nervous tissue, for it is in all probability one of the ganglia of the autonomic system. On the other hand, the secretions of the medulla are definitely endocrine in nature and have metabolic effects that are not always correlated with the nervous activity. The secretions of the medulla, *epinephrine* and *norepinephrine*, thus are mediators of the autonomic system and at the same time are endocrine substances.

HORMONES OF THE ADRENAL MEDULLA

Epinephrine was the first of all the hormones to be characterized. The second hormone of the medulla, norepinephrine, was not isolated from the adrenal until 35 years later, although it was synthesized about the same time as epinephrine. The hormones are produced in chromaffin cells of the gland, and each is stored in a different granule. The relative secretion rates appear to vary from time to time, as will be discussed. The chromaffin cells are differentiated from neuroblasts and are named from the brown color that results when they are stained with chromic acid. The hormones are synthesized in part by the mitochondrial fraction of the cells and probably stored in a bound form, since injection of intact mitochondrial particles results in about one-fifth the total activity of the extract, whereas injection of lysed granules supplies the total activity. Acetycholine is the mediator of splanchnic nerve stimulation of the gland, which releases hormone from the bound form in granules.

Biological synthesis of each of the hormones is well documented. Incubation of medullary segments with carbon-14-labeled phenylalanine or tyrosine results in the synthesis of epinephrine. The process probably proceeds through Dopa (dihydroxy-phenylalanine) and dopamine (the corresponding dihydroxy-phenylanine) to norepinephrine. The norepinephrine is methylated on its amine N to produce epinephrine (Figure 8.1). This process can be readily demonstrated *in vitro*. The hormones are extremely labile and are readily oxidized to *adrenochromes*, colored by-products of degradation of the molecule. The synthesis of epinephrine from norepinephrine can be demonstrated by indirect experiment.

When the adrenal medullary hormones are synthesized, they are stored in granules in the gland. They are released by a dissolution of the granules mediated by Ca++ under acetycholine stimulation. It is interesting that different factors will change the secretion rate. Epinephrine is released under stressful situations when the stress is "known," while norepinephrine is released under unexpected "unknown" stresses. Under normal conditions, the gland releases about 80 percent norepinephrine and 20 percent epinephrine, but this ratio

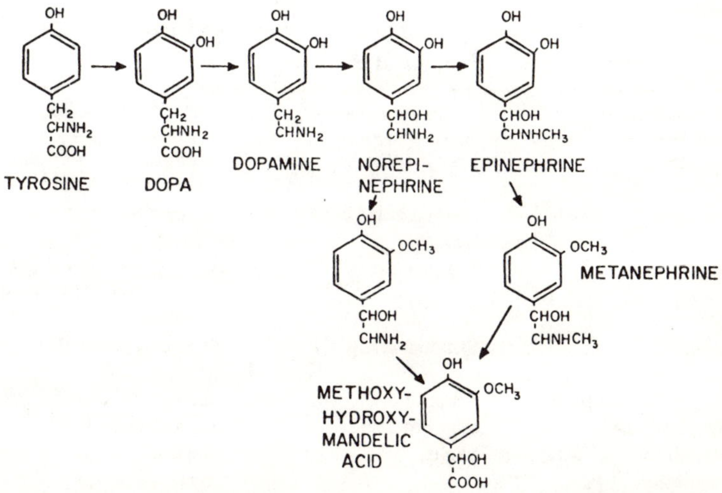

Figure 8.1. The biosynthesis of the adrenal medullary hormones.

may be reversed. If an adrenal gland is stimulated by the splanchinc nerve and the venous effluent analyzed for epinephrine, the first output is about 60 percent epinephrine. Continued stimulation results in a decrease in epinephrine to 25 percent or less of the original output with a sustained norepinephrine output. Furthermore, if a methyl donor such as methionine is furnished the gland, the output of epinephrine can be sustained.

Extremely small amounts of the medullary substances circulate in the blood at any one time, and this has led to statements that the hormones are secreted only under stress. Von Euler claims that about 0.015 micrograms per kilogram of body weight per minute is normally secreted and that this rises rapidly to 1.1 micrograms per kilogram per minute upon stimulation of the splanchnic nerves. The hormones are rapidly destroyed by the liver and probably by nerve endings, where the material acts as a transmitter substance.

Activity of Medullary Hormones. Epinephrine and norepinephrine vary in their action on different organs as shown in Table 8.1. As an example of species specificity, the ratio of activity of epinephrine to norepinephrine is about 75:1 on the rat uterus, whereas in the pregnant cat uterus the ratio is about 0.1:1, a difference of 750 times. It is often difficult to differentiate between the metabolic activity of the two amines, which may represent true hormonal action, and their

Table 8.1. Effects of epinephrine and norepinephrine on various organs of the body.

Activity	Norepinephrine	Epinephrine
Heart *in situ*	Bradycardia—increased force	Tachycardia—increased force
Heart *in vitro*	Tachycardia—increased force	Tachycardia—increased force
Blood vessels	Vasoconstriction	Vasoconstriction in skin, viscera; vasodilation in muscle
Glands (sweat, salivary, etc.)	Stimulates slightly	Stimulates strongly
Oxygen consumption	Little effect	Marked increase
Glycogenolysis	Slight increase	Marked increase
Adrenal ascorbic acid depletion	Slight	Marked
Muscle lactic acid	Slight increase	Marked increase

activity as autonomic mediators. The present concept is that norepinephrine is the substance liberated at postganglionic adrenergic nerve endings, and that epinephrine is produced only by the adrenal medulla. Epinephrine has by far the greater influence on metabolism.

Epinephrine, when administered exogenously, is able to trigger the anterior pituitary, probably through the hypothalamus, to cause the release of ACTH, and, as suggested by the ability to block ovulation, it is concerned with normal release of FSH and LH. Present evidence implicates 1-DOPA, rather than epinephrine itself, as the active agent in the body. Many of the metabolic activities attributed to epinephrine may be due to the triggering action of this substance on the anterior pituitary. This is true, for example, of the hyperglycemic activity, which may be mediated through adrenal steroids as well as through the direct activity of epinephrine itself.

Aside from its effects on the organism as a neural transmitter, epinephrine has many metabolic actions, most of which are far more potent than norepinephrine (Table 8.2). When epinephrine is administered to an animal, there is a rapid release of glucose by glycogenolysis from the liver with a subsequent rise in blood sugar (Figures 8.2 and 8.3). This comprises one of the adjustments of the body to a stressful situation.

Epinephrine also produces a sudden and dramatic rise in production of blood lactic acid, which quickly returns to normal. As the lactic acid returns toward normal, liver glycogen rises, which indicates that the process of

$$\text{muscle glycogen} \rightarrow \text{lactic acid} \rightarrow \text{liver glycogen}$$

has occurred to restore the liver glycogen depleted by the first action of epinephrine. As a result of the combination of processes, the liver glycogen drops rapidly at first, then gradually rises to a level greater

Table 8.2. Relative actions of epinephrine and norepinephrine on various sites.

Site of Action	Action	Epinephrine	Norepinephrine
Vascular system	Vasoconstriction	+	++++
Central nervous	General excitation	++++	0
Liver	Glycogenolysis	+++	+
Hypothalamus	Pituitary stimulation	+++	±
Muscle	Lactate production	+++	0

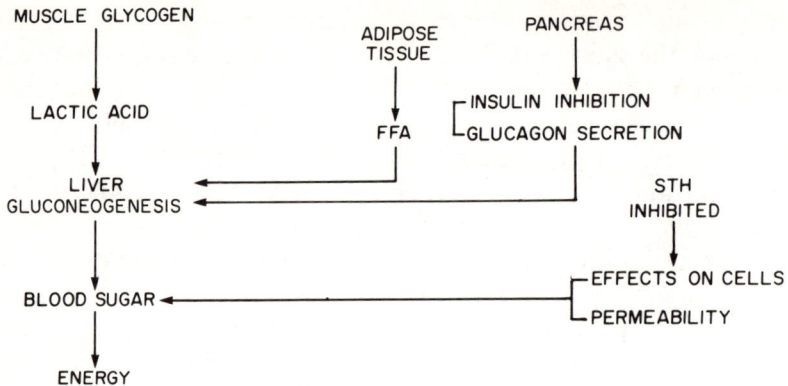

Figure 8.2. The generalized effects of epinephrine on metabolic functions.

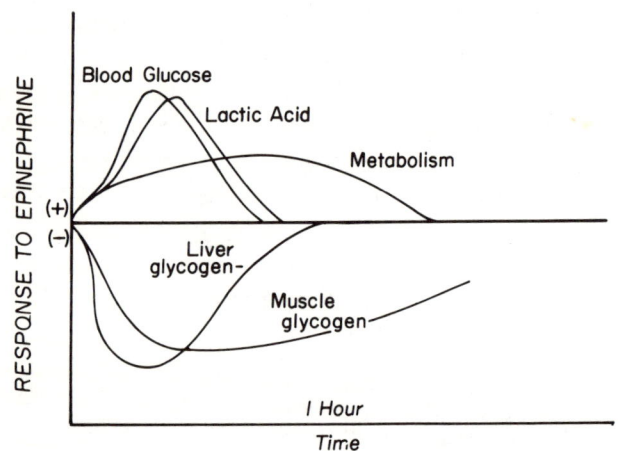

Figure 8.3. A schematic diagram of the time course of the events outlined in Figure 8.2.

than normal. Also, a decrease in muscle glycogen occurs, which could be predicted from the preceding scheme.

The site of action of the hormone occurs at the stage where glycogen is converted to glucose-1-phosphate (Figure 8.4). Epinephrine increases the rate of this reaction, and it can be demonstrated that the level of hexosephosphates rises in muscles treated with epinephrine.

Fatigued muscle appears to have smaller amounts of the phosphorylase enzyme present, and it may be that one of the factors producing fatigue is a decrease in the conversion of glycogen to hexosephosphate.

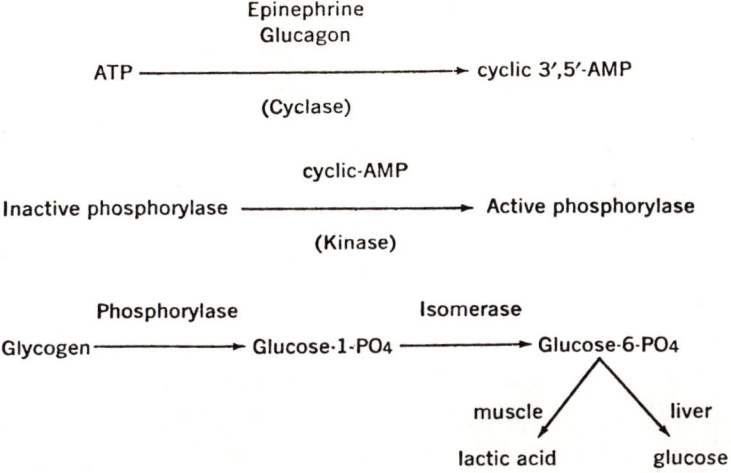

Figure 8.4. The sites of action of epinephrine in glucose metabolism.

At any rate, epinephrine stimulates the activation of phosphorylase, which may prevent the onset of fatigue.

The epinephrine mechanism provides an admirable example of the checks-and-balances system in the endocrine regulation of homeokinesis. When insulin is present in excess, the blood sugar is decreased, the decreased blood sugar triggers the adrenal medulla, and epinephrine is released. The epinephrine then causes the glycogen to be broken down to glucose, which raises the blood sugar back to normal. A rapid secretion of somatotrophin in responses to hypoglycemia to restore the blood glucose to normal also occurs to complement the adrenergic response.

There is another site of action of epinephrine in the muscle. It is a well-known observation that epinephrine causes vasodilation in the muscle, whereas norephinephrine causes vasoconstriction. The accumulation of metabolites such as lactic acid, when produced by increased epinephrine output, may lead to a passive dilation of the blood vessels, overriding inherent vasoconstrictor activity; however, the activity of norepinephrine as a vasoconstrictor, which does not produce metabolites to any great extent (about one-tenth of the activity of epinephrine), is not masked by metabolic effect. As a broad generalization, epinephrine has longer-term metabolic effects, whereas norepinephrine has a shorter-acting, largely cardiovascular effect on the organism.

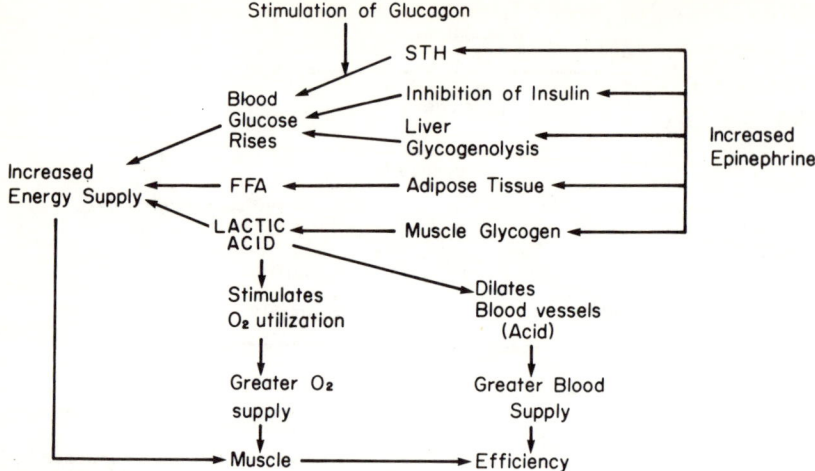

Figure 8.5. The effects of increased production of epinephrine under stress to provide energy sources.

Figure 8.5 illustrated clearly the many metabolic functions that are performed by epinephrine. The direct action of epinephrine on fat breakdown, glycogenolysis, and inhibition of insulin secretion, coupled with the stimulation of GH secretion and changes in blood supply, all help to provide the energy to meet stress.

There does not appear to be a demonstrable feedback control of the adrenal medulla. Response is to a neural trigger induced by stress and is designed so that the organism can respond better to that stress, although end results are often contradictory.

Hypofunction of the adrenal medulla is unkown as a specific syndrome. If excised adrenal tissue is transplanted to another site, the cortex (but not the medulla) will regenerate. Under these conditions, there are no demonstrable abnormalities. One reason may be that norepinephrine and perhaps some epinephrine are produced by sympathetic nerve cells as transmitting agents.

Hyperfunction, on the other hand, is a serious disease. If a tumor of the secreting type, *pheochromocytoma*, develops in the gland, the effects are a combination of the metabolic and nervous functions of the gland: hyperglycemia, extremely high blood pressure, and other symptoms of excessive sympathetic stimulation.

Assay of Catecholamines. Because of the clinical importance of the adrenal medulla, many attempts have been made to provide a satisfactory assay for the hormones. The most common assays now in use involve measurement of the blood pressure of the dog, the contraction of muscle (rectal cecum of the chicken), and other biological assays. All of these assays are somewhat limited because norepinephrine and epinephrine give different responses and are present in variable amounts in serum or urine. In addition, the assays vary widely in accuracy since many predisposing factors can affect the results. Within the last few years, methods have been developed for the fluorometric assay of the hormones after their separation by chromatography from blood or urine, and chemical conversion to strongly fluorescing derivatives of adrenochrome. The resulting values are called "catecholamine levels" to point up the nonspecificity of the method. Although prior chromotography is a great improvement, none of the methods is completely satisfactory because many materials, including catecholamines both related and unrelated to the adrenal catecholamines, fluoresce or otherwise interfere with the determination. The results obtained in different laboratories vary widely. Mass spectroscopy now offers much better methods.

In the early 1920's, Walter Cannon proposed that two types of material circulated in the bloodstream, *sympathin I* and *sympathin E*, producing, respectively, the inhibitory or excitatory effects noted in some organs. With the physiological discovery of norepinephrine, many workers presumed this new material to be sympathin E, while epinephrine was supposed to be sympathin I. Although there is some superficial evidence of this separation, it is now believed that the effects of stimulation and inhibition are produced by different types of receptors in the end organ, which respond to epinephrine or norepinephrine in different ways.

References

Hingerty, D. and A. O'Boyle. *Clinical Chemistry of the Adrenal Medulla*. Springfield, Illinois: Charles C Thomas, 1972.

Vane, J. R. *Adrenergic Mechanisms*. Boston: Little, Brown, 1960.

9
Calcium Metabolism: Parathyroid Hormone and Thyrocalcitonin

PARATHYROID HORMONE

The parathyroid glands are essential for life. In the majority of individuals, there are four to six small yellowish-red bodies, lying in the dorsal portion of the thyroid. The total weight of these glands is approximately 100 milligrams. The parathyroids have an abundant blood supply and do not appear to be stimulated by the meager nerve supply.

Close examination reveals that each gland consists of two types of cells: the *chief cell*, usually considered to be hormone-producing, and the *oxyphil cell*, containing acidophilic cytoplasm. In the young, only the chief cells are present; the oxyphil cells appear with advancing age, possibly being derived from the former. The cells produce a blood-calcium–*elevating* polypeptide hormone, which has been designated as parathyroid hormone (PTH). The hormone has been obtained in reasonably pure form only within the last few years (previous preparations are now estimated to have been less than 1 percent pure). Data of Harold Rasmussen indicate that the active hormone C is a polypeptide with a molecular weight of about 8,500, but con-

Table 9.1. Characteristic of bovine parathyroid hormone.

Parathyroid Hormone	Molecular Weight	Units/mg	Amino-Acid Residues
A	3,800–5,200	750–1,250	33
B	7,000	1,600	62
C	8,450	3,200	84

siderable activity remains in two still smaller products, A and B, split from the larger molecule (see Table 9.1).

Further work with gel filtration purification has suggested that PTH is a polypeptide of 84 amino-acid residues, with alanine as N-terminal and leucine as C-terminal, having a molecular weight of 8,500. Biological activity is about 3,000 international units/ milligram.

Some evidence suggests that Pro-PTH is formed in the cell, cleaved to an 84-amino-acid residue (PTH), which is stored in the secretory granules; finally, a further cleavage may occur in the blood to a hormone of perhaps 32 amino acids that is biologically active.

In recent years, evidence has accumulated for a blood-calcium–*lowering* hormone produced by the thyroid-parathyroid complex. Originally called calcitonin, it has been renamed *thyrocalcitonin* (TCT) to indicate its thyroidal origin. It will be discussed later in this chapter.

THE BONE

There are two types of cells concerned with the metabolism of bone. The *osteoclasts*, which resorb bone by removing both the calcium phosphate and protein matrix, and *osteoblasts*, which synthesize new bone. A third cell type, the *osteocytes*, also serve in calcium metabolism and appear to be a rapid response mechanism as opposed to the longer response time of the osteoclasts. The mechanism of resorption is of particular interest because the dissolution of a calcium (apatite) matrix is a remarkable feat. The calcium must be dissolved, moved across the cell, and secreted into the blood to be used or excreted by the kidney. This process is difficult to imagine, and several theories have developed involving active transport, complexing of calcium, number and activity of osteoclasts, and thus resorption of bone. The action of PTH is mediated by c-AMP.

The osteoblasts synthesize long polypeptide chains, which are then cleaved, and three strands are interwoven to form pro-collagen. The pro-collagen is transported to cell membranes and secreted. Several chains are linked together to form collagen. The calcium phosphate is deposited in the interstices along the fibers. Mitochondria may be necessary to mobilize the calcium for deposition, and ATP is required for the energetics of the process. Nucleation sites then form, and the solid apatite crystals are deposited. The two processes of bone resorption and deposition are closely interrelated. Bone is continuously remodeled as a necessary process independent of control of serum calcium. Normally, the process is in balance, and osteoblastic and osteoclastic activity are equal.

CONTROL OF CALCIUM LEVEL

The general form of the control of Ca^{++} level by the combination of factors is illustrated in Figure 9.1, and this is related to the calcium

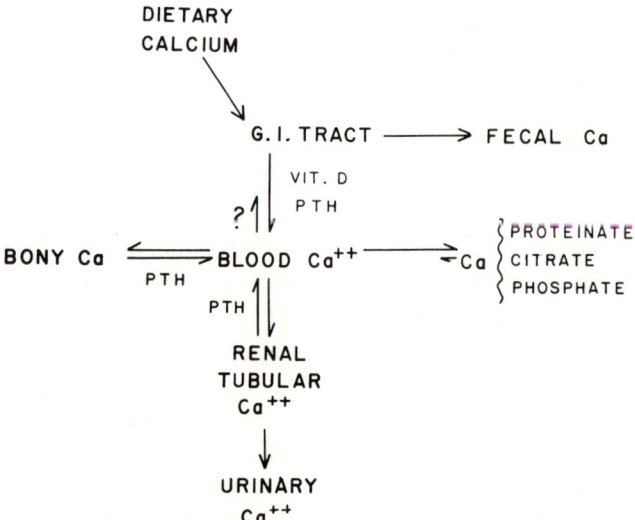

Figure 9.1. A diagram illustrating some of the metabolic interrelationships of calcium in the body, indicating sites of action of parathyroid hormone (PTH) and thyrocalcitonin (TCT).

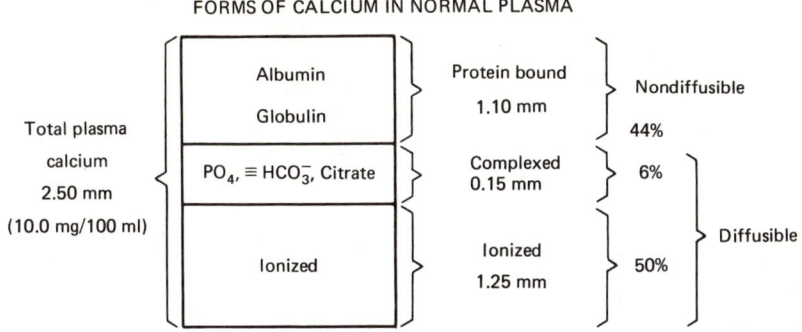

Figure 9.2. The situation of calcium in the plasma indicating the free (active) and the bound (inactive) forms.

levels in the plasma (Figure 9.2). It is apparent that the control of body calcium must take into account many factors; absorption from the gut, bone distribution, kidney activity, and the parathyroid and thyroid glands. As already mentioned, the controlled level is the *free* Ca^{++} ion rather than the large amount of calcium fixed to protein or bone.

Transport of Ca^{++} through the gut is largely determined by the presenting concentration of the ion. Uptake is decreased by phosphate. PTH appears to have some little effect in increasing calcium absorption.

The kidneys perform two functions: reabsorption and an excretion of calcium. The kidney usually resorbs nearly all of the calcium filtered at the glomerulus through active transport. PTH increases absorption probably thru a c-AMP–mediated process. At the same time, PTH *inhibits* the phosphate-transport mechanism and *reduces* the resorption of phosphate with a corresponding increase in excretion.

These relationships are presented in the control diagram in Figure 9.3, which illustrates the action of PTH on kidney, bone, and plasma concentration.

The bony skeleton takes up calcium and lays down bone through poorly understood mechanisms. The ability of GH to stimulate bone formation has already been mentioned, and thyroid, insulin, and estrogen also stimulate bone formation, whereas cortisol and PTH depress it. Vitamin D has little effect on deposition of bone. On the other hand, vitamin D, PTH, and TCT do affect resorption. TCT decreases resorption, whereas PTH increases it and vitamin D inhibits resorption.

146 INTEGRATION AND COORDINATION OF METABOLIC PROCESSES

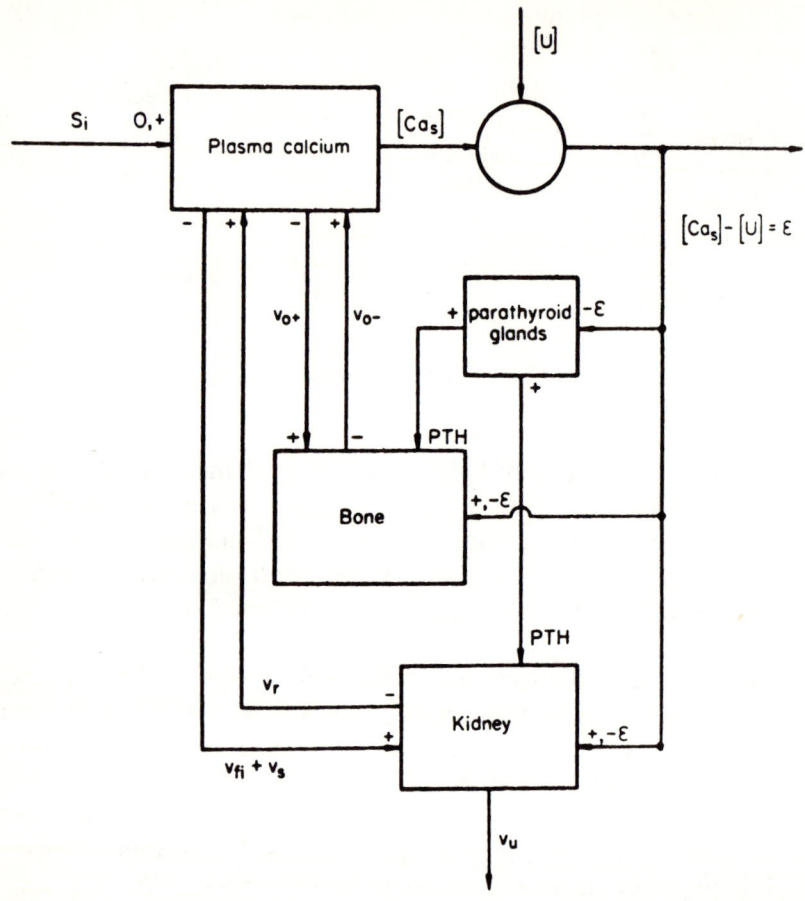

Figure 9.3. A simplified diagram of Figure 9.4 showing the main control points and the feedback in a general scheme of calcium metabolism. (Taken from Brown and Gann, *Engineering Principles in Physiology*, Academic Press, New York, 1975, with permission.)

The overall control of serum Ca^{++} appears to be a balance between PTH and TCT secretion (Figure 9.4). Figure 9.5 attempts to outline the quantitative terms of the whole control system and ties together the effects on the liver, kidney, and gut to control serum calcium.

Present evidence suggests that both PTH and TCT are secreted continuously, and the plasma Ca^{++} level is the result of balance between the two hormones (Figures 9.6 and 9.7).

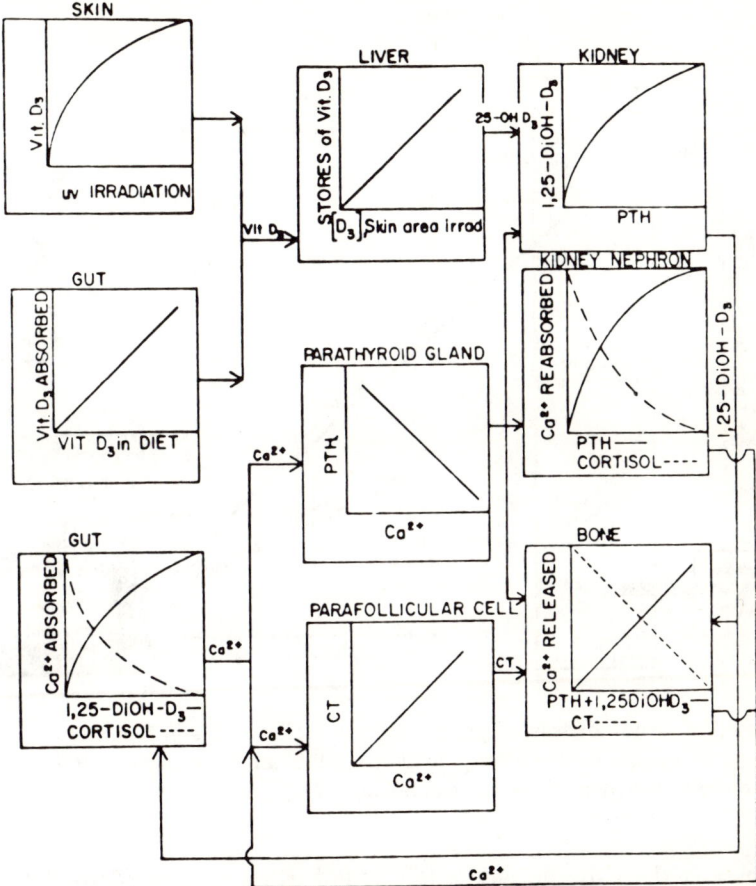

Figure 9.4. The control of calcium metabolism indicating the relationship between PTH, TCT, and vitamin D on bone, kidney, liver, and gut. (Taken from Kline, *Biological Foundations of Biomedical Engineering*, Little, Brown, Boston, 1976, with permission.)

VITAMIN D

One of the major controls in calcium metabolism is vitamin D. Vitamin D exists in several forms, including D_3, cholecalciferol, which arises from irradiation of 7-dehydrocholesterol in the skin. D_3 is formed in the skin or absorbed from the gut, which is then transported to the liver where it is converted to 25-OHD_3. Then it is

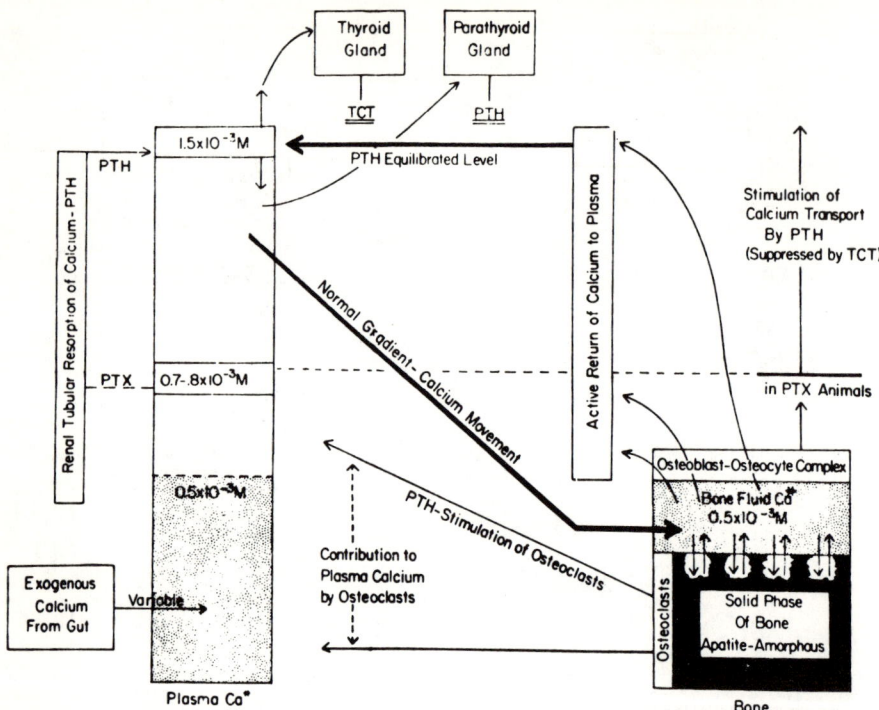

Figure 9.5. Another way of presenting much of the data in Figure 9.2 in such a way as to present quantitative data in concentration. (Taken from *Handbook of Physiology*, American Physiological Society, Washington, with permission.)

transported to the kidney where it is further converted to the 1,25-dihydroxy cholecalciferol (1,25-OHD$_3$). This is the most potent metabolite and increases Ca^{++} absorption in the gut (Figure 9.8). It is not known whether D$_3$ affects calcium or phosphate reabsorption of the kidney tubule to any physiological extent, although small effects can be measured. In the parathyroidectomized animal, the 1,25 OHD$_3$ is not made; 24,25 OHD$_3$ is made instead, indicating some effect of PTH on renal function. The 1,25 OHD$_3$ acts on the intestine to increase calcium-absorption deposition. The receptor in the intestine, and probably in bone, is a cytosol receptor with nuclear activity, similar to steroid receptors. Vitamin D has interesting effects in bone because, in the presence of PTH, it appears to be able to increase bone resorption and then to lay down new bone,

CALCIUM METABOLISM 149

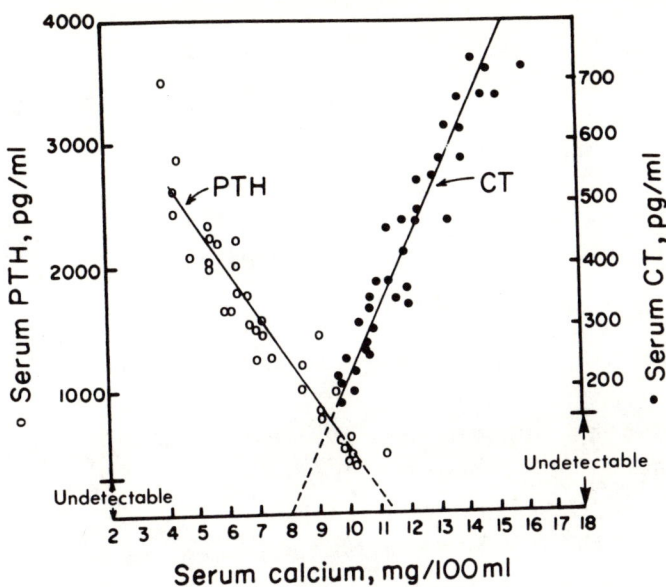

Figure 9.6. Concentrations of CT and PTH against serum calcium demonstrating the reciprocal relationship with a "set point" at the normal plasma level. (From Arnaud, C. D., et al., *J. Clin. Invest.* 50 [1971] : 21.)

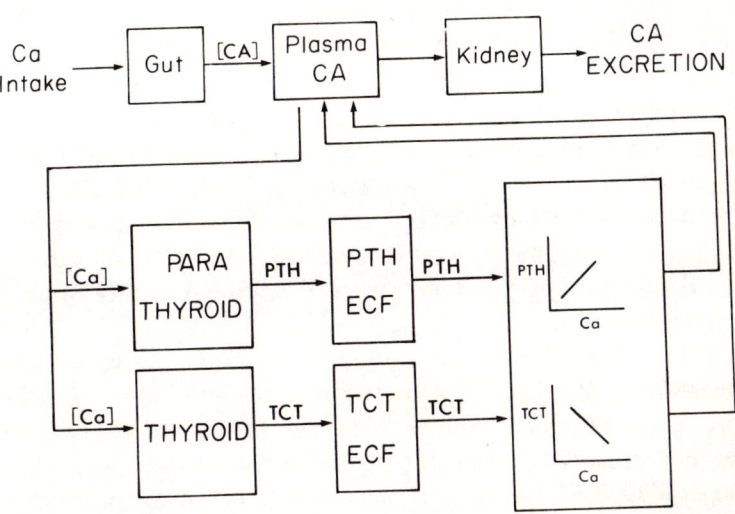

Figure 9.7. A control diagram of the data in Figure 9.6 demonstrating the parallel control system.

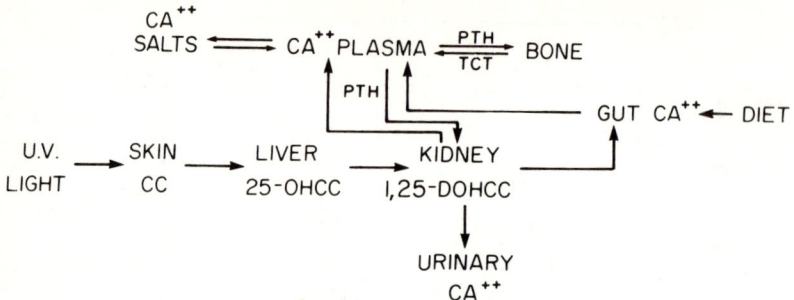

Figure 9.8. The relationship of vitamin D to absorption of calcium including formation of 1,25, DOHCC from skin irradiation and kidney activity.

thus increasing turnover, although results are not yet totally convincing.

CALCIUM AND PHOSPHATE METABOLISM

Examination of the distribution of calcium in the human body reveals a total of about 1,000 grams of calcium, 99 percent of which is located in the bony skeleton. The blood serum and extracellular fluid calcium, consisting of about 0.06 percent (600 milligrams) of the total, is solely concerned in the homeokinesis of calcium ion level through the mechanism of the parathyroid hormone secretion. This fraction, which performs all of the metabolic activity, is backed up by the labile pool of calcium of about 500 grams. The great bulk of calcium present in the bones and teeth is so far removed from any blood vessels that it is not available to body processes, although recent evidence obtained with Ca^{45} suggests that bony calcium is more readily exchanged than previously realized. The dynamic balance of body calcium is illustrated in Figure 9.9, which clearly shows the interchanges that occur.

Ionized calcium (or calcium complexed with citrate) is excreted by the kidney. Extensive reabsorption of calcium ion occurs in both the proximal and distal tubules. The administration of parathyroid hormone decreases calcium excretion by the kidney by decreasing the rate of plasma clearance of calcium compared to the glomerular filtration rate. This may occur even in the presence of a high plasma calcium resulting from calcium-loading and at a time when the clearance might well be expected to increase. Conversely, parathyroidec-

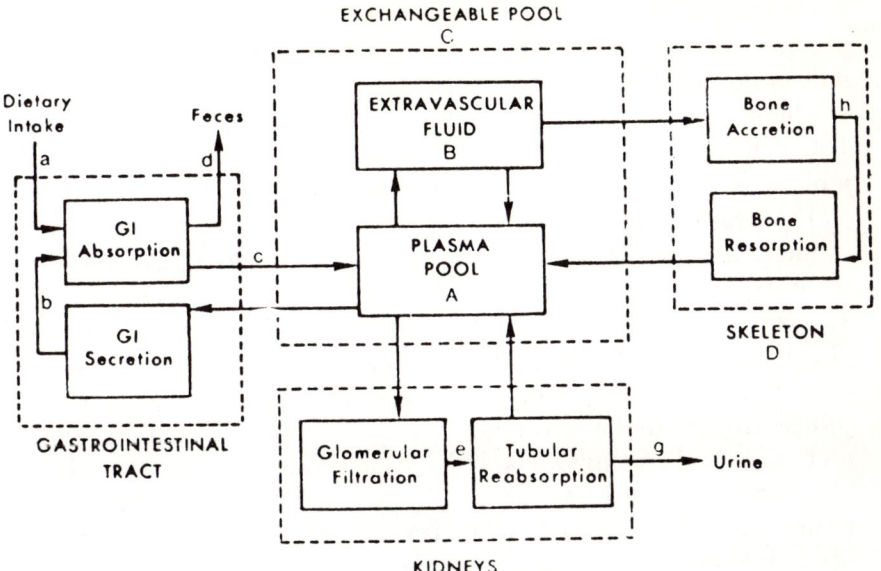

Figure 9.9. The interchanges between the major spaces of the body with regard to calcium.

tomy increases the urinary calcium by increasing the clearance, that is, by causing less reabsorption of the ion. Increased plasma ionized calcium in the absence of injected PTH may result in an increase in the renal clearance of calcium. There appears to be no limit to the clearance of calcium under normal conditions when the serum calcium is elevated.

The effect on the kidney has been well demonstrated by Talmadge who found that administration of PTH resulted, first, in a fall in urinary Ca^{++} under influence of the hormone and, second, in an increased excretion of Ca^{++} as the plasma Ca^{++} reached high levels. The secondary rise is probably due solely to the increased filtration of calcium by the kidney as a result of increased bone resorption and increased plasma Ca^{++} levels. The reverse is true in parathyroidectomized animal in which the lowered T_m results in a sudden increase in Ca^{++} excretion followed by a drop in plasma Ca^{++}; later, the urinary Ca^{++} excretion decreases as plasma level falls.

Under normal conditions, about 80 percent of the body's phosphorus is in the bone. The remainder is in the tissues as a constituent of protoplasm and in the body fluids. The most labile form of phosphorus is that combined with organic molecules (as adenosinetriphosphate, phosphocreatine, and phospho-enolpyruvate) to provide the high-energy phosphate bonds that are necessary for the metabolic processes of the body. Under normal conditions, phosphorus is present in the plasma at a level of about 2.4 milligrams per 100 milliliters, of which 12 percent is protein-bound, 45 percent is ionized, and 43 percent is complexed with other ions.

The present evidence suggests that only the inorganic fraction is influenced by parathyroid hormone. The kidney tubule is able to reabsorb only limited amounts of phosphate ion, and a very definite T_m exists. It is clear that parathyroidectomy decreases urinary phosphate excretion, and most workers agree that injection of PTH increases it. In the dog, unilateral renal artery injection of PTH will result in an increased excretion of phosphate on the injected side, with no change in the contralateral kidney. Because of the limited tubular phosphate reabsorptive capacity, there has been a tendency to assume that PTH causes tubular secretion of phosphate, but there is little direct evidence for such a concept.

Because of the fundamental importance of phosphorus in cellular metabolism, many attempts have been made to find an action of parathyroid hormone on uptake of phosphate into cells, on permeability of cells to phosphate, or on combination of phosphate with cellular components. Although suggestions of such effects have been noted, no definite proof exists.

In discussing the physical chemistry of calcium phosphates in the body, it has always been customary to emphasize the importance of the ion product; i.e., ($Ca^{++} \times PO_4$). When the product of the concentration of calcium and phosphate exceeds a certain maximal value, known as the solubility product, precipitation of calcium phosphate will occur. Since bone is largely calcium phosphate, the tendency toward calcification *in vivo* has often been presented exclusively in terms of the plasma calcium and phosphate. Normal values are about 10 and 5 milligrams per 100 milliliters of plasma, respectively, yielding a product of 50. When either calcium or phosphorus falls to such an extent that the product drops below 30, rickets (inadequate bone formation) may develop. Elevation of the product above 60 indicates a tendency toward soft-tissue calcification. It should be emphasized that such a simplified scheme is satisfactory for clinical observations, but interpretation must take into account not only the actual concentration but also the activity coefficients of the ions, which may vary markedly under different conditions of hydration, pH, and so on.

Although this has furnished a convenient framework for empirical presentation, the usefulness of such a concept in biological systems has become very limited. Calcification is known to occur at low Ca × P values.

At the other extreme, it is obvious that the Ca × P product in plasma is several times higher than that possible in simple solution, demonstrating that there are other factors at work that make this oversimplified version quite inadequate.

One influence on the ion product is protein that, as has already been mentioned, is capable of binding a wide variety of materials, including calcium. McClean and Hastings pointed out many years ago that calcium salts and protein in the physiological pH range formed a weakly dissociated calcium proteinate. They described what has been the only practical method of determining the calcium ion level in a biological fluid by using the perfused isolated frog heart as a test object. Since the strength of the heartbeat is directly proportional to the calcium ion concentration, the effect of perfusion of an isolated heart with an unknown solution is matched with that of a known solution. By this method, it was found that about 4.7 milligrams per 100 milliliters of plasma was ionized, of the total calcium of 10.0 milligrams per 100 milliliters. Ultrafiltration experiments demonstrate that about half (5 milligrams per 100 milliliters discrepancy between 4.7 milligrams ionized and 5.0 milligrams per milliliters diffusable calcium) may represent calcium citrate. Important new data can be expected from use of the newly introduced calcium ion electrodes.

There are, of course, important functions of calcium in the body other than control of excitability. Calcium ions are also involved in blood coagulation and membrane permeability (including that of blood vessels). Calcium is an integral component of the hydroxy- and fluoroapatite mineral structure of the bones and teeth. Since both the calcium and phosphate withdrawn from bone under parathyroid hormone action are in the ionic form, it is logical to assume that the process of mineralization involves ionic form. Although phosphorus is intimately involved in calcium metabolism, it also participates in other quite different functions, including buffering of body fluids and energy transfer in intermediary metabolism through formation of such high-energy phosphate compounds as adenosinetriphosphate and phosphocreatine. These aspects should be pursued by reading biochemistry and physiology texts.

METABOLIC EFFECTS OF THE PARATHYROIDS

When the parathyroids are removed from a normal susceptible animal (such as a goat or dog), the serum calcium decreases and the serum phosphorus increases. The urinary phosphorus decreases markedly. After an early hypercalciuria, there may be either no change or a decrease in excretion of urinary calcium. The animal first becomes listless and fails to eat. Muscular twitching starts, which within several hours develops into frank convulsions that can be blocked by curare, thus indicating a nervous origin. Eventually, death results from spasm of the skeletal muscles concerned with respiration.

Before death, events usually occur in cycles. In the presence of a lowered serum calcium, a spasm develops, the muscles are forced to do more work, carbon dioxide and lactic acid accumulate, and this excites the respiratory center to increase respiration. The increased respiration, in turn, increases the carbon dioxide output through the lungs, makes the blood more basic, lowers calcium ionization, and increases the irritability. As respiratory muscles become spastically paralyzed, carbon dioxide rises faster than it can be eliminated, lactic acid is produced by anaerobically contracting muscles, and the pH of the blood becomes more acidic. This raises the concentration of calcium ion, and the convulsion stops. As the pH again rises and the calcium ionization decreases, the cycle starts again. If the disease continues, the spasms occur more frequently until recovery is impossible.

An early alteration in kidney function following parathyroidectomy is the decrease in urinary phosphorus excretion. According to one theory, the decrease in excretion of phosphorus leads to increased retention and higher levels in the plasma; this, in turn, affects the solubility product of calcium phosphate, and the calcium level falls. A lowered calcium level in the plasma results in decreased urinary calcium, and phosphate excretion occurs; however, careful analyses by Munson and others show that there is no increase in serum phosphate until long after the drop in calcium is apparent. This circumstance has emphasized the concept of a direct PTH action of the equilibrium between bone calcium and calcium in the extracellular fluid, as will be discussed later.

When PTH is injected, the changes are, in general, reversed. There is increased serum calcium, decreased serum phosphorus, increased urinary phosphorus, and usually increased urinary calcium. The degree of elevation of serum calcium is proportional to the dose of PTH within limits. If injections of large amounts of hormone are continued for many days, there is marked lethargy due to decreased neuromuscular irritability from the elevated calcium levels. There are pronounced calcification of soft tissues and the formation of renal calculuses, which often lead to death from renal failure. That the bones are the ultimate source of the extra calcium is proved by their extensive demineralization. The great difficulty of achieving satisfactory regulation of plasma calcium by means of injected PTH emphasizes the delicacy of the intrinsic homeokinetic mechanisms.

There is a close relationship between calcium-phosphorus metabolism and the remainder of the endocrine system, even though a specific action of PTH is not always manifest. The gonadal hormones have profound effects on the deposition of bone. Testosterone increases bone size, matrix formation, and retention of calcium and phosphorus. Estrogens have a stimulating effect on osteoblasts and accelerate bone maturation and formation. In this connection, the parathyroid of the hen should be investigated further, because hens are able to deposit a considerable fraction of their body weight per day as calcium into the shell of eggs and into the egg itself. On a low-calcium diet, the hen can mobilize 25 percent of its total weight for eggs. The parathyroid has an effect on other tissues. Many hormone actions are mediated by CA^{++} ions at cell walls and in the cytoplasm.

The hormones of the adrenal cortex have a catabolic effect on protein with a resultant decrease in matrix formation in bone, leading to osteoporosis and excess calcium in urine. The thyroid hormone increases the basal metabolic rate of most cells and causes specific maturation of bone. In the absence of the thyroid, bone growth is decreased. In hyperthyroidism, there is less laying down of protein in the bone matrix, and osteoporosis develops. Growth hormone in excess has a somewhat similar action.

THYROCALCITONIN

In contrast to the blood-calcium–raising effect of parathyroid hormone, secreted in response to lowered calcium levels, evidence accumulating in the last few years has indicated the existence of a rapid calcium-*lowering* hormone called *calcitonin*, secreted by the cells of the thyroid. Purification of a polypeptide of low-molecular-weight protein prepared from parathyroid-free thyroid tissue has yielded the most active calcitonin preparations, with a chain of 32 amino acids.

TCT causes a rapid decrease in serum Ca^{++}. The effect is produced by an inhibition of bone resorption. The serum phosphate is also lowered immediately. Both of these effects are enhanced by increased excretion of Ca^{++} and phosphate by the kidney. TCT also has some effects in inhibiting Ca^{++}-*reabsorption* by the kidney.

PTH and TCT relationships have already been discussed. However, the gastrointestinal hormones, gastrin and cholecystokinin, may also have a feedback control. When soluble Ca^{++}-containing substances are introduced into the gastrointestinal tract, the release of hormones (glucagon, gastrin, and cholecystokinin from the gut) produce prompt secretion of TCT.

References

Aurbach, G. D. et al. "Hyperparathyroidism: Recent Studies." *Ann. Int. Med.* **79** (1973): 566–581.

DeLuca, H. "The Kidney as an Endocrine Organ for the Production of 1.25-Dihydroxy-Vitamin D2, a Calcium-Mobilizing Hormone." *New England Journal of Medicine* **289** (1973): 359–365.

10
The Pancreas

The pancreas is an organ of both exocrine and endocrine function. It lies in the curve of the duodenum and as an exocrine organ supplies various digestive enzymes to the intestinal contents. Enzyme production occurs in the acinar tissue, which comprises 99 percent of the weight of the pancreas. Lying embedded in the acinar tissue are clusters of endocrine cells, which are easily distinguished histologically. The islets of Langerhans (named for Paul Langerhans, a German physician, who first described them) produce at least two separate secretions. One secretion, insulin, is a well-known hormone; the other, glucagon, has only recently had its endocrine role completely established (Figure 10.1).

Although *diabetes mellitus*, the disease associated with lack of insulin, was well known in its overt form by the ancient Egyptians and Romans, it was not actually demonstrated until 1899 when Von Mering and Minkowski removed the pancreas from a dog and showed that diabetes resulted from the operation. Later, it was found that although ligation of the pancreatic duct resulted in atrophy of the acinar tissue, it did not produce diabetes, and no changes resulted in the islet tissue. In 1922, Banting and Best succeeded in obtaining extracts of such duct-ligated glands, which were effective in depancreatized dogs. Soon afterwards, Collip produced, from bovine pancreas extracts, insulin solutions suitable for treatment of human diabetics.

The severity of the disease following removal of the pancreas

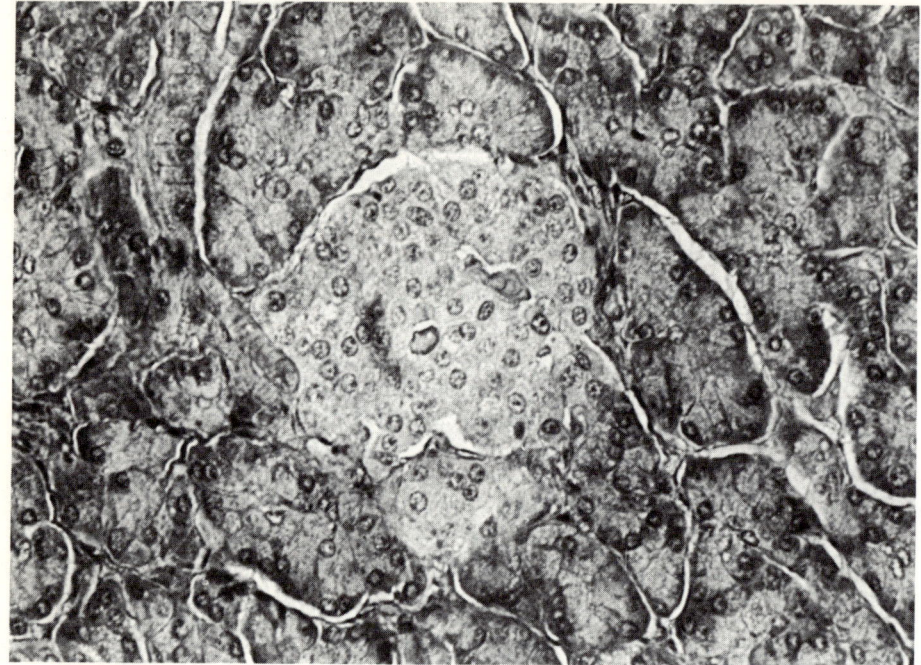

Figure 10.1. A histological section of the pancreas showing the light-colored endocrine bodies buried in a mass of exocrine tissue.

appears to vary with species; carnivorous animals develop more severe symptoms than the herbivorous groups.

CARBOHYDRATE METABOLISM

The individual cells of the body function in the normal situation by burning carbohydrates to provide the energy to carry out the synthetic and degradative processes, which together are called *metabolism* (Figure 10.2). The supply of glucose thus becomes a critical factor in metabolic processes. Usually, the glucose supplied to the cells arrives from the bloodstream where it is maintained by the liver at a relatively constant level of about 100 milligrams per 100 milliliters of blood by the combined process of production of glucose from glycogen and gluconeogenesis. Extrahepatic cells, in turn, utilize glucose in the formation of glycogen, protein, and fat, and oxidize it to carbon dioxide and water to provide the energy to carry out the

THE PANCREAS   159

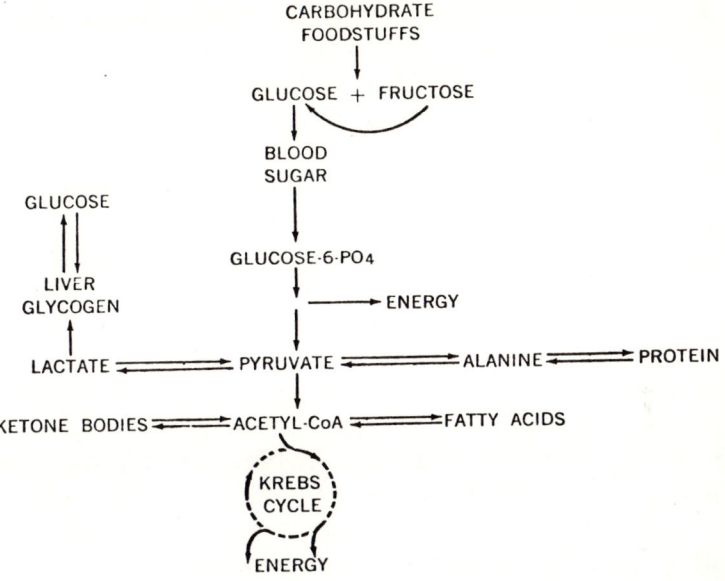

Figure 10.2. A rough schematic to indicate the overall pattern of carbohydrate metabolism, which is influenced by insulin.

other processes, as well as any specialized functions such as muscular contraction and secretion. The entire process is so regulated that the blood sugar in the normal organism remains relatively constant.

The maintenance of the constant blood glucose supply to the cells is achieved in large degree by the liver. This organ is able to convert its glycogen to blood sugar if the level of the latter falls and is able to form glycogen from blood sugar and lactic acid when the levels of these materials rise. The rates of these processes are governed by several hormones (Figure 10.3). The uptake of sugar from the gut is accelerated by thyroid hormone; the breakdown of glycogen to

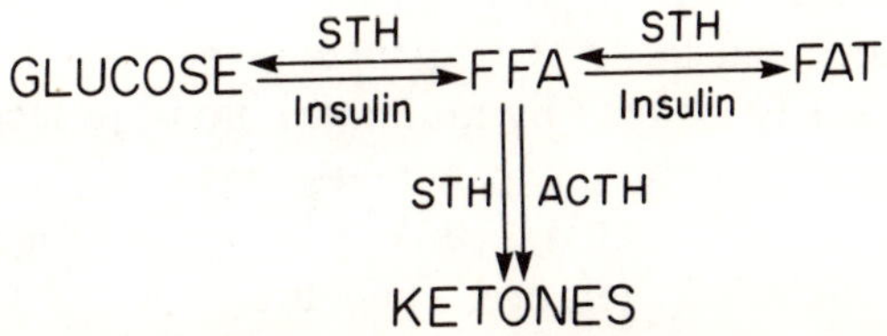

$$GLUCOSE \underset{Insulin}{\overset{STH}{\rightleftarrows}} FFA \underset{Insulin}{\overset{STH}{\rightleftarrows}} FAT$$

$$\underset{KETONES}{\overset{STH \;\; ACTH}{\Downarrow}}$$

Figure 10.3. The interconversion of the carbohydrate fat and protein in metabolic processes indicating the interrelationship among the endocrine secretions.

glucose in the liver with concomitant changes in muscle is stimulated by epinephrine; increase in blood sugar through gluconeogenesis is brought about by the action of the adrenocortical steroids; and inhibition of glucose utilization apparently occurs through the action of pituitary growth hormone. The precise minute-to-minute regulation of the blood sugar level is brought about by secretion or inhibition of secretion of insulin, which is delicately tied in with all of the processes of carbohydrate movement outlined previously.

INSULIN

The major hormones secreted by the pancreas are insulin and glucagon. Insulin is a polypeptide with a minimal molecular weight of 6,000 and an isoelectric point of 5.3. Insulin readily forms crystals containing zinc, although the exact location of the metal ion is not known. Zinc insulinate is useful both for purification and for formation of an insoluble complex with protamine to yield "depot" insulin. The activity of an insulin preparation is compared to a standard using a bioassay method, which is usually the fall in blood sugar level of rabbits or the production of hypoglycemic convulsions in mice.

The brilliant work of Sanger in England culminated in elucidation of the complete structure of the insulin molecule. As shown in Figure 10.4, it consists of one chain of 21 amino acids (chain A) with an internal disulfide bridge between two cysteines and connected through two other cysteine-S-S-cysteine bridges to the B-chain of 30 amino acids. Both chains have been synthesized, but joining them through the proper disulfide links has proved difficult.

The hormone varies among species, but all variations are confined to the amino acids between the disulfide linkages. Because of the small structural differences, all purified insulins have the same activity, and insulin from one species is fully active in other animals. There is some immunological response, and occasional instances of insulin resistance can be traced to species-specific protein reactions. Insulin can be easily assayed by radioimmunoassay techniques.

Insulin is produced in the pancreatic beta cell as a prohormone with three polypeptide chains linked together (Figure 10.4). On secretion, the C-chain is removed, and the A and B active chains are secreted. The prohormone is packaged in the beta cell in granules in the Golgi apparatus along with inactive proteases, which digest away the C-chain before secretion. The pancreas normally contains about

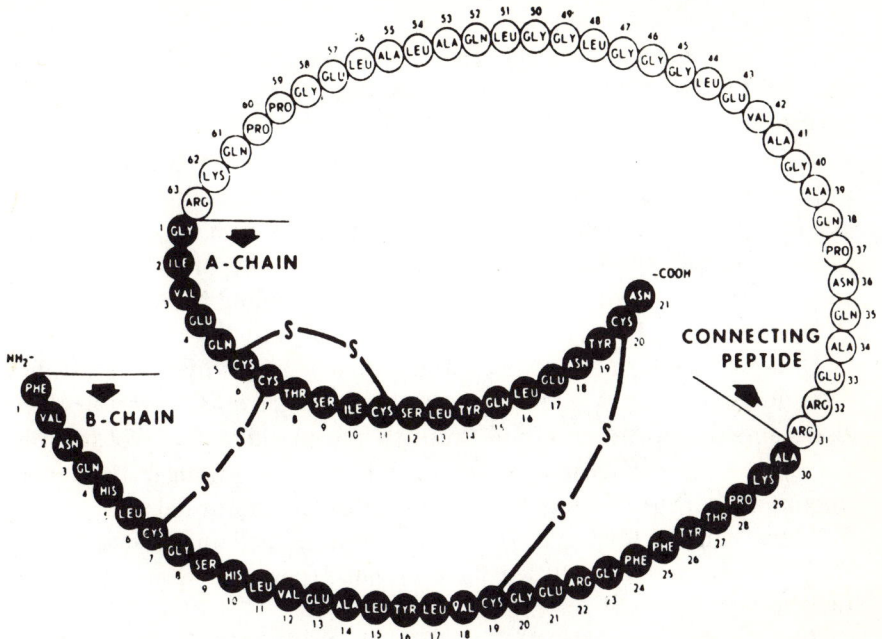

Figure 10.4. The prohormone of insulin, showing the A- and B-chains (insulin) joined by the inactive C-chain together with the sulfide bridges connecting the chain.

400 units of insulin. Normally, about 40 units per day are secreted. The protease in the beta cell granules are activated by c-AMP. Ca^{++} is necessary for the process, and an influx of Ca^{++} can be noted when the cell secretes.

The hormone is rapidly destroyed in the blood. The half-life of intravenously injected insulin is about 1 hour, at least partly because it is rapidly destroyed by *insulinase* of blood and other tissues, although the specific nature of such enzyme activity is still vigorously debated. Tissue-binding of insulin is also an important factor, as will be discussed later. Some of the difficulty in elucidating such reactions resides in the very difficult assay of the extremely small amount of the hormone (0.001 unit/milliliter) present in blood and tissues under normal conditions.

Insulin Activity: Effects of Insulin Lack. Removal of the pancreas results in a variety of changes, partly endocrine and partly exocrine. We will concentrate here upon the effects related to a deficiency of secretion from the islet tissue that can be repaired by administering extracts of such tissue. The first and most immediate effect is that of hyperglycemia, with blood sugars in the range of 300 milligrams per 100 milliliters of blood. The actual value depends upon diet, and lower values are obtained upon fasting. When the blood sugar exceeds the renal threshold (i.e., when the capacity of the renal tubule to reabsorb glucose is exceeded), glycosuria occurs. In the severe diabetic, the total exogenous glucose intake may be excreted in the urine along with the additional sugar supplied by the processes of gluconeogenesis.

Under normal circumstances when glucose is administered, insulin secretion is initiated as the arterial blood sugar concentration level rises, and the hormone rapidly returns the blood sugar level to normal. In such a *glucose-tolerance curve*, the blood sugar rises to a maximum within about 1 hour and is returned to normal within 2 to 3 hours. In the diabetic, insulin function is inadequate; the blood sugar rises to a very high level and remains there for a long period of time.

The diabetic exhibits other metabolic abnormalities. The respiratory quotient (RQ) is the ratio of carbon dioxide produced by the organism to the molecular oxygen taken up in the same interval of time. Carbohydrate foodstuffs that are burned with a greater requirement of oxygen for a given production of carbon dioxide will have a higher RQ than those substances (fat) that require less oxygen to oxidize the same molecular weight of material. On a theoretical basis, RQ's higher than 1.0 would signify transformation of carbohydrate into fat. In actual practice, these are usually artifactual, being obtained under conditions of net loss of carbon dioxide from the body's bicarbonate buffer pool, as during strenuous exercise. The normal person usually has an RQ of about 0.8, which represents the metabolism of mixtures of foodstuffs including carbohydrate, fat, and protein, the latter with an RQ of 0.84. In contrast, the RQ of the diabetic is usually about 0.7 indicating that fat is being burned almost exclusively. In addition, the diabetic usually excretes large amounts of ketone bodies, a by-product of fat metabolism (Figure 10.5).

One interpretation of the foregoing information is that the diabetic is unable to utilize normal amounts of glucose and that fat is burned as a source of energy. Glucose continues to be formed from

THE METABOLISM OF FATS

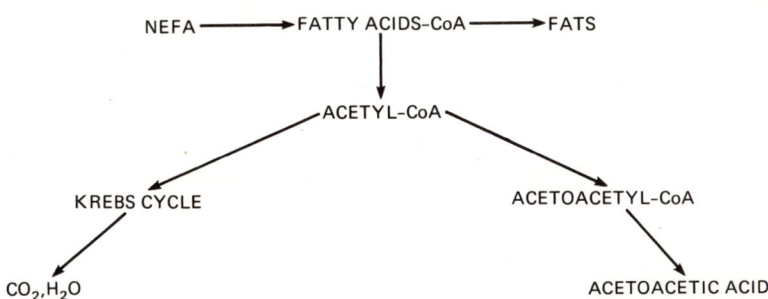

Figure 10.5. The normal pathway of fat metabolism is through the Krebs cycle, but when the cycle is overloaded, as may occur in diabetes, more actyl groups are forced into the pathways leading to acetoacetate formation (ketone bodies).

amino acids and is lost in the urine. As much as 5 to 7 grams of nitrogen per day may be lost as a result of the breakdown of protein in this way. The nitrogen balance of the diabetic is directly related to the amount of insulin supplied him and the exogenous carbohydrate metabolized as a consequence. Diabetics supply the energy to maintain life by breaking down fat and protein from their bodies. The ketone bodies produced as a by-product of fatty-acid and amino-acid metabolism may rise from the normal value of 1 to 2 mg/100 ml to 10 or even 100 mg/100 ml, and the excretion of ketone bodies in the urine may increase from negligible values to as much as 20 grams per day. The loss of energy by this means is not excessive (160 calories), but the loss of sodium may be very high. Ten grams of ketone bodies excreted at pH 5, where the pK of the acid is also about 5, would require 50 meq of sodium per day for partial neutralization. This loss of cations eventually results in acidosis.

As the metabolic changes occur during the development of diabetes, a characteristic picture emerges. Diabetes has often been called the "*poly*-disease." The failure to furnish material for energy to the cells results in overeating, *poly*phagia; the excretion of sugar in the urine results in high urine volume, *poly*uria; and the loss of fluid results in thirst, *poly*dipsia. These effects are summarized in Figure 10.6.

It should not be concluded that the body uses no glucose in the absence of insulin. The well-fed diabetic is able to store some glyco-

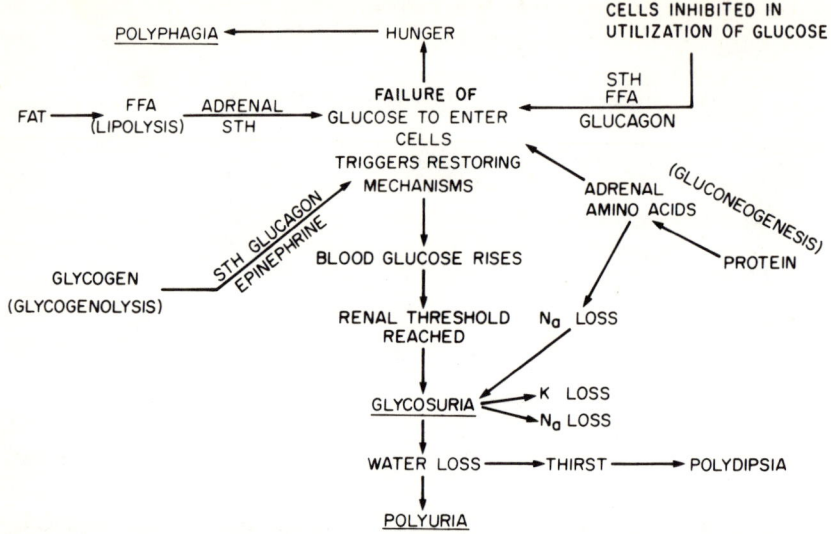

Figure 10.6. The overall effect on body metabolism of diabetes. Note the generalized effects far beyond that of carbohydrate metabolism alone.

gen in the liver from an elevated blood sugar. In the diabetic hepatectomized animal, the blood sugar falls continuously, indicating some utilization of glucose in the periphery. If the concentration of glucose is raised, utilization is increased, suggesting a mass-action effect. The outstanding effect of insulin may be to enable glucose to be used by the cell at a lower blood level than without the hormone. Furthermore, the central nervous system clearly does not require insulin in order to metabolize glucose.

There appears to be two kinds of glucose transport into the cell. There is a *demand transport,* which occurs when some feedback signal, perhaps a product of glucose metabolism, stimulates the transport of glucose as usage by the cell rises. There is also a *supply transport,* which occurs only because the concentration difference between the blood and the cell promotes diffusion or transport through an unsaturated transport mechanism. Insulin appears to increase the capacity of the supply system. The transport system is coupled to the cellular sodium pump. When the sodium pump is blocked with ouabain, glucose transport increases. The sodium pump is dependent only on constant energy supply; therefore, a failure of the pump triggers a greater input of energy in the form of glucose. The transport of glucose is also inhibited by fatty acids. This may be important in starvation and lead to the sparing of glucose for those organs that must have it, such as the brain.

In addition to the alterations of carbohydrate, fat, and protein metabolism, other changes occur in the metabolic pathways. The diabetic may excrete 100 grams of sugar per day in the urine. This amount of solute requires a considerable quantity of water, because the kidney is unable to raise the urine osmotic concentration much above 1,200 milliosmols per liter. As a result, the urine volume increases. If the sugar were excreted in a 2 percent solution, the kidney would be required to produce a minimum of 5 liters of urine per day. The renal loss of salts and other materials that are filtered and not completely reabsorbed also increases the urine volume. A severe diabetic may lose 36 meq of sodium and 20 meq of potassium per day more than a normal individual. The former represents the sodium equivalent of 250 milliliters of body fluid and indicates dehydration. The loss of potassium would represent 2,000 milliliters of extracellular fluid because of its low potassium concentration and consequently must indicate the release of potassium from cells being broken down because of the demand for gluconeogenesis.

Site of Action of Insulin. Many years of evidence suggested that insulin in some way permitted the utilization of carbohydrate by the organism. In the absence of insulin, most cells of the body were believed to be unable to utilize carbohydrate and relied on other sources of energy. When insulin was provided, the ability of the cells to utilize sugar returned. This "underutilization" explanation of diabetes was opposed by the contrasting opinion that insulin regulated glucose production, especially from fat. This theory considered diabetes due to "overproduction" of glucose, without any defect in oxidation. It is now realized that many aspects of both concepts are true, since there clearly is glucose overproduction, primarily from protein, along with the diabetic's greatly diminished ability to utilize carbohydrate for energy.

A major site of insulin action on carbohydrate metabolism must be in the extrahepatic tissues of the body since the hormone is effective in the hepatectomized animal. This observation was extended by Gemmill, who found that glucose was taken up by the rat diaphragm incubated *in vitro* and that such uptake was accelerated by insulin. Considerable quantities of glycogen could also be deposited under the influence of insulin.

Cori and coworkers suggested that the site of insulin action was at the level of hexokinase in the phosphorylative scheme of carbohydrate breakdown. Using various tissue preparations, they reported that insulin could remove an inhibition imposed on the hexokinase system by certain anterior pituitary extracts. Such an observation could not explain all of insulin's activity, since it was much more active in the total absence of the pituitary. In addition, other laboratories were not consistently able to confirm the basic observations.

The most critical series of experiments on the site of insulin action was reported by Levine. In a diabetic dog infused with glucose, the sugar occupied a space approximately equal to the extracellular fluid. When insulin was administered, the available space for glucose distribution suddenly increased. Only one explanation was possible—that insulin increased cellular penetration of glucose. Further work demonstrated that all sugars with the same steric configuration on the first three carbons (d-galactose, l-arabinose, d-xylose, and d-glucose) were taken up at increased rates when insulin was given, despite the fact that arabinose and xylose were not metabolized in the body (Figure 10.7).

A change in some permeability or transport function is implied, although there is still no clearly formulated process by which the insulin membrane effect can be explained. Apparently the brain, which does not require insulin in order to utilize glucose, possesses a different membrane-transport mechanism. Under high blood sugar

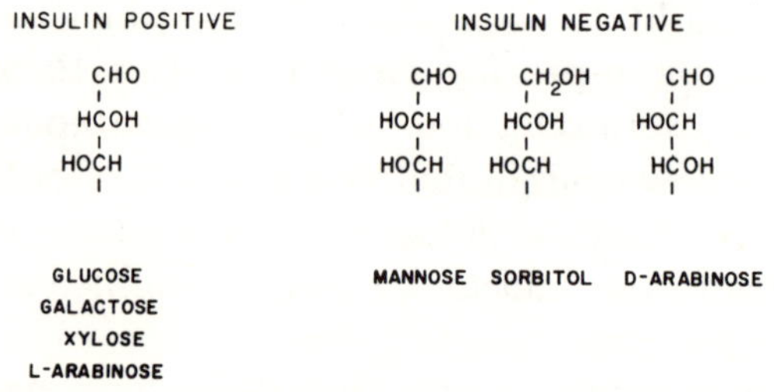

	INSULIN POSITIVE	INSULIN NEGATIVE		
	CHO | HCOH | HOCH |	CHO | HOCH | HOCH |	CH$_2$OH | HCOH | HOCH |	CHO | HOCH | HCOH |
	GLUCOSE GALACTOSE XYLOSE L-ARABINOSE	MANNOSE	SORBITOL	D-ARABINOSE

Figure 10.7. The structures of the sugar molecules, which are influenced by insulin. Only the first three carbon atoms are shown, as the configuration of the other atoms is not concerned in this reaction. Only those molecules with a structure identical to glucose on the first carbon atoms are able to penetrate the cell wall at an increased rate under the influence of insulin.

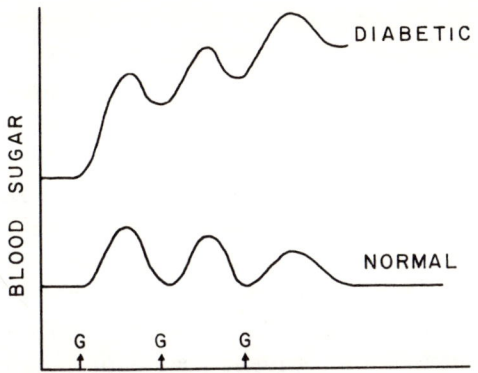

Figure 10.8. The response of normal and diabetic individuals to successive doses of glucose administered at G. Note the increasing blood sugar of the diabetic as contrasted to decreasing response in the normal person.

levels, all tissues of the diabetic animal appear to be able to utilize small amounts of glucose, which is probably due to a mass-action effect. This work has been extended in many directions, including a return by Stadie to study of insulin action on Gemmill's isolated diaphragm preparation. Stadie was able to show that insulin was bound in an almost irreversible form to the tissue protein prior to its effect on permeability.

It should be noted that the effect of insulin on membrane permeability is not the only possible action of the hormone. It has been found, for example, that insulin accelerates the uptake of P^{32} into organic phosphate compounds, and the thought remains that insulin may have some direct effect upon glucose breakdown, perhaps at the site of two-carbon-chain entry into the Krebs cycle. There is also the yet unexplained phenomenon of increased fat production from carbohydrate, along with reports of increased oxygen consumption by various tissue preparations when insulin is added, but these bear only a dubious relationship to insulin activity in intact cells.

Control of Insulin Secretion. Another problem is the control of insulin secretion. It has been known for many years that administration of glucose will cause a definite response in the blood sugar consisting of a rapid rise followed by a decline to former levels. If a second dose is administered as the first hyperglycemic phase begins to wane, the second response is not as large as the first. A third dose will give a still smaller response. It has been suggested that the secretion of insulin stimulated by the first glucose is still in progress when subsequent doses are given, with a resulting decreased level of hyperglycemia. This may be confirmed by repeating the same experiment in the diabetic in whom each dose causes a greater response in the blood sugar than did the previous dose (Figure 10.8). It has also been demonstrated that in animals on a high-carbohydrate diet, the amount of insulin in the pancreas may decrease to about one-tenth of its normal value, indicating that insulin is secreted in response to the blood sugar level. The conclusive experiments were performed by Foa, who perfused the effluent pancreatic blood from one dog into a second animal. When the first animal received glucose, the blood sugar of the second animal fell, indicating insulin secretion by the pancreas of the first dog in response to the glucose level.

The present evidence favors the view that the control of insulin secretion is mediated directly through the bood sugar level. A rise in blood sugar stimulates the beta cells of the pancreas, which in turn produce insulin to return the blood sugar to normal. The process is a modification of the feedback systems previously described for the other hormones; that is, there is no evidence at present that the control of insulin secretion is governed by hypothalamic or pituitary pathways. It is possible that the feedback may *not* be glucose but a metabolic product of glucose. Use of radioimmunoassay techniques show that the average cell contains about 11,000 receptors for the insulin molecule. These receptors are on the cell plasma membrane, and insulin therefore acts through a second messenger. Brain, kidney, intestine, and the red blood cells contain few receptors and utilize glucose without the need for insulin. Cortisol decreases the ability of the cells to bind insulin and adrenalectomy will restore the binding capacity.

Insulin apparently acts to increase the transport mechanism, which is relatively nonspecific. All sugars with approximately the same steric configuration are facilitated in their transport by insulin, but none of them except glucose can feed back as a control. This again suggests that metabolites may be the actual feedback.

Insulin is probably secreted from the cells in a biphasic response. The administration of glucose will trigger an immediate release of insulin (within 7 minutes), which decreases even if the glucose administration is continued. The initial rapid response is followed by

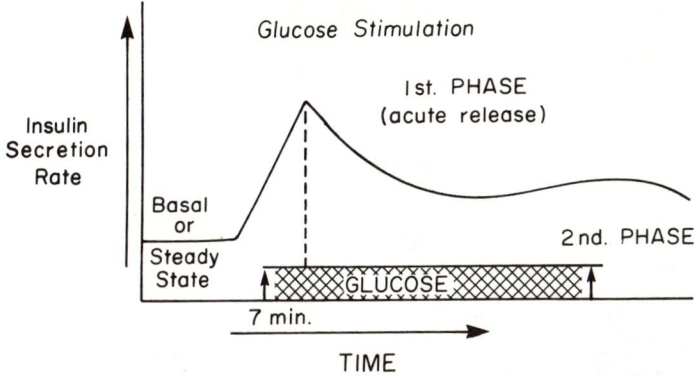

Figure 10.9 The biphasic pattern of secretion of insulin with time with administration of glucose.

a prolonged increase in insulin secretion (Figure 10.9). It has been proposed that this represents a release of "last-in, first-out" hormone, which may be more available followed by the dissolution of further granules. If glucose is administered in single divided doses, each dose causes an increased secretion, whereas the diabetic is unable to secrete insulin on demand and his or her blood sugar rises rapidly.

Innervation of the Pancreas. For a long period, the pancreas was believed to function with a direct feedback from the plasma glucose level to the beta cells. This idea was based largely on the fact that a transplanted pancreas without a nerve supply functioned very well.

However, the pancreas is well innervated. It has adrenergic receptors and cholinergic receptors. Bolivian experiments have demonstrated that when food is introduced into the stomach, a response secretion of insulin occurs *before* the gastrointestinal secretagogues appear, which are known to stimulate insulin production. These facts have been placed in a control diagram, Figure 10.10. Although these effects are real, the actual influence on the minute-to-minute circulating insulin levels are probably slight.

One interesting speculation has come about because of the interest in the nervous stimulation of the pancreas. Figure 10.9 demonstrates the well-known insulin secretion response to a continued administration of glucose. It has been suggested that the first sharp peak results from release of a small, labile, "first-in, first-out" pool of insulin, and

170 INTEGRATION AND COORDINATION OF METABOLIC PROCESSES

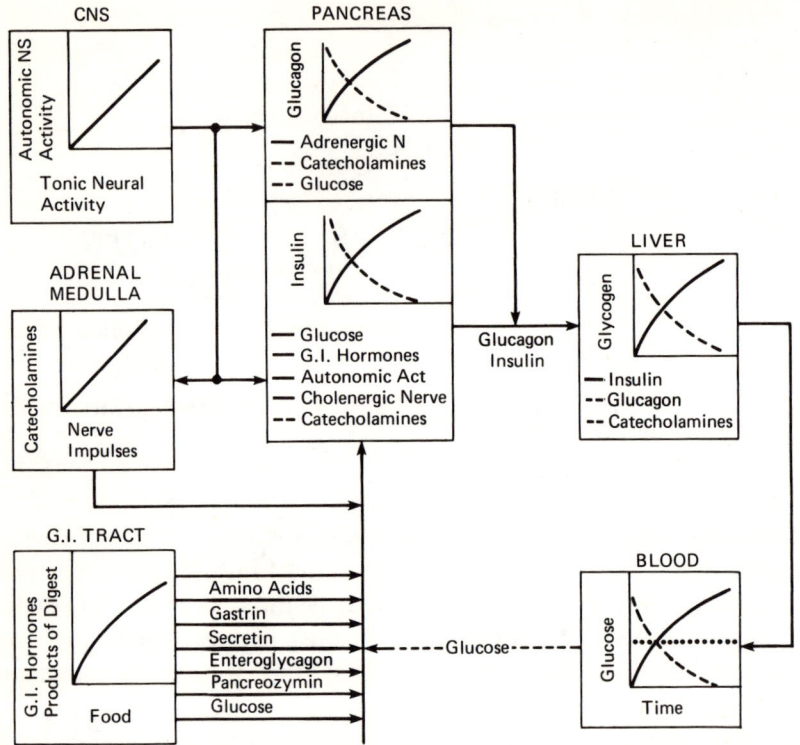

Figure 10.10. The control of insulin secretion. (Taken from Kline, *Biological Foundation of Biomedical Engineering*, Little, Brown, Boston, 1976, with permission.)

that the long sustained rise comes about from the release of a larger, more stable insulin pool. Epinephrine may serve as a mechanism to transfer insulin from the small to the large pool and thus retard its release.

Other Insulin Effects. Insulin has effects in the body other than the simple control of carbohydrate metabolic processes. It has been demonstrated that insulin is required in order to obtain the maximum effect of either growth hormone or the androgens on retention of nitrogen. Insulin is necessary for the action of growth hormone but the reverse is not true. This may explain the nutritional experiments demonstrating that a certain number of calories in the form of carbohydrate must be available to the cell in order to obtain satisfactory deposition of protein and anabolism of nitrogen. In addition, insulin will cause a decrease in the plasma amino nitrogen concentration independent of its effect on carbohydrate metabolism. This may be due to an increased cellular amino-acid uptake, since insulin produces a markedly increased uptake of α-amino isobutyric acid, even though this unnatural amino acid cannot be utilized further by the cell. Recent observations show that insulin increases amino-acid incorporation into tissue proteins.

Interrelationships of the Pancreas. It should be emphasized that hypo- and hyperglycemia can be produced by mechanisms not directly involving insulin excess or lack. The administration of adrenocortical steroids, for example, increases gluconeogenesis and produces hyperglycemia or *steroid diabetes*, which is only distantly related to the pancreatic form. It is true that such hyperglycemia will stimulate production of insulin from the pancreas; if continued, it may exhaust the islets and result in semipermanent diabetes. Epinephrine will cause a temporary hyperglycemia. Some individuals have a low renal threshold, spill sugar in the urine at low plasma levels, and develop "spontaneous" hypoglycemia independent of insulin secretion (renal diabetes).

In addition to the hyperglycemia produced by underproduction of insulin, pancreatic tumors may develop, which produce more insulin than normal with a resulting hypoglycemia. This must be differentiated from the condition of a vigorous hepatic removal of blood sugar resulting in hypoglycemia. The latter condition tends to occur after normal insulin secretion; however, various types of glycogen-storage diseases are known to occur in which the storage of carbohydrate during a plethora is not matched by its withdrawal when necessary to maintain the blood sugar.

The effects of insulin on fat and protein metabolisms are demonstrated in Tables 10.1 and 10.2, and Figure 10.11. Insulin operates in these two systems much as it does in carbohydrate metabolism, by controlling processes around a "set point." It is also obvious that insulin has an effect on both catabolism and anabolism, and the overall effect must be taken into consideration in predicting results.

The pituitary plays a complex role in carbohydrate metabolism. The animal treated with anterior-pituitary extract becomes insulin-resistant (i.e., more insulin is required to produce a given change

172 INTEGRATION AND COORDINATION OF METABOLIC PROCESSES

Table 10.1. The influence of insulin excess or deficit
on control of fat metabolism.

(Redrawn from Tepperman, *Endocrine Physiology and Metabolism*, Year Book, 1974.)

Insulin +		Insulin −
	Synthesis	
↑	1. Glucose uptake pyrophosphate formation 2. Glycenophosphate formation 3. Pyurate dehydrogenation 4. Citrate transport 5. Triglyceride formation	↓
	Oxidation	
↓	1. Lypolysis 2. Free fatty acid release 3. Polnutyl C_0A formation	↑

in blood sugar), while the hypophysectomized animal is highly insulin-sensitive. A considerable portion of this effect is a result of the gluconeogenesis previously mentioned as resulting from stimulation of the adrenal cortex by ACTH; however, this is not the entire picture. GH inhibits glucose utilization by the tissues, which, in turn, produces a type of *pituitary diabetes*. GH increases the demand

Table 10.2. The influence of insulin excess of deficit
on control of protein metabolism.

(Redrawn from Tepperman, *Endocrine Physiology and Metabolism*, Year Book, 1974.)

Insulin +		Insulin −
	Synthesis	
↑	1. Amino acid uptake 2. Protein formation 3. Ribosome activity	↓
	Catabolism	
↓	1. Amino acid release from muscle 2. AA in plasma 3. Gluconeogenesis	↑

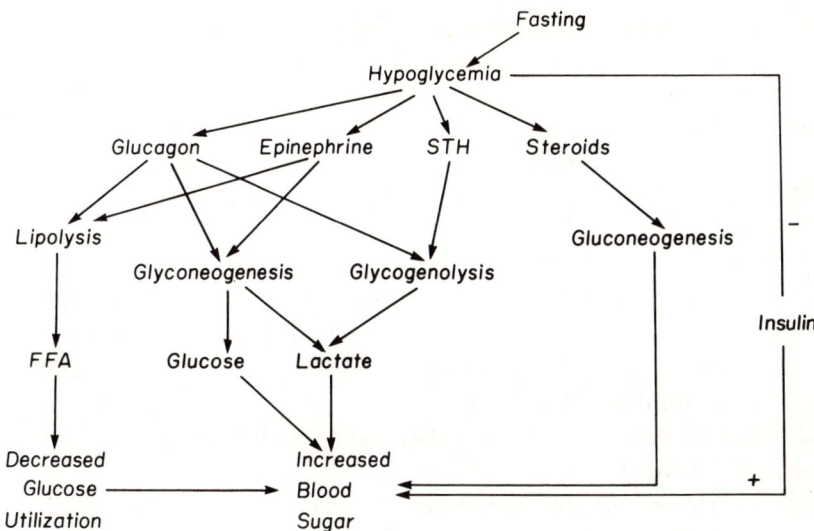

Figure 10.11 The effects of hypoglycemia on the endocrine system indicating the sum of the mechanisms that act to restore the blood glucose levels.

of the body for insulin, probably due to anabolic activity, and the pituitary diabetes reflects a relative, rather than an absolute, insufficiency of insulin. This is borne out by observations that extra insulin will decrease the diabetogenic effect of GH. Injection of GH to hypophysectomized-pancreatectomized dogs (Houssay animals) exacerbates the diabetes in the complete absence of insulin, indicating the independent action of the two glands on the utilization of glucose.

Insulin behaves differently in the starved animal. As energy sources decrease and the liver begins breakdown of fat to ketone bodies, the effect of insulin on the cell is decreased so that the ability of a given dose of insulin to lower blood is markedly reduced. At the same time, the brain, which has depended on glucose, develops an ability to metabolize ketone bodies. This conditioning is reflected in cellular function. When glucose is suddenly administered to a starving system, it is unable to utilize it, and glycosuria results.

Insulin improves amino-acid transport into cells and decreases FFA mobilization and increases FFA deposition. The small fat cells of young animals are more insulin-sensitive than the large cells of older animals. It could be postulated that cells contain equal numbers of receptors, and these are in lower concentration on the surface of the big fat cells.

Insulin promotes protein synthesis at the translational (ribosome) level and inhibits gluconeogenesis in the liver. Most of the actions have already been summarized in Figure 10.5, which presents the effect of diabetes on the cell as opposed to the presence of insulin discussed here.

The overall metabolic relationships are summarized in Figure 10.11. The control system in Figure 10.10 indicates clearly the relationship among the pancreas, kidney, adrenal medulla, and the gastrointestinal tract. Figure 10.11 tries to represent the pathways of metabolism and the insulin point of action of these pathways. Tables 10.1 and 10.2 clearly illustrate the effects of insulin on fat and protein metabolism, which of course are closely tied to the effects of carbohydrate metabolism, which we have already discussed. Figure 10.10 attempts to put together a control diagram illustrating the influence of all of these factors on the blood sugar.

Oversecretion and Undersecretion. Because of the nature of the action of insulin, both oversecretion and undersecretion may be dangerous. With excess insulin, the blood sugar decreases to extremely low levels, and the cells of the nervous system are unable to obtain energy for normal function. As a result, hypoglycemic shock develops, involving convulsions and coma. The obvious means of obtaining relief is to administer glucose to restore the blood sugar. In undersecretion, the body is unable to metabolize the glucose presented to it. Hyperglycemia results in glycosuria and dehydration, and the preponderant fat oxidation causes ketosis, acidosis, and electrolyte depletion. The net result is diabetic coma, which requires immediate treatment with insulin, fluid, electrolyte, and other measures to return the metabolic pattern toward normal.

ORAL HYPOGLYCEMIC AGENTS

One of the major annoyances in the treatment of diabetes is the administration of insulin that must be given by injection, which may result in induration, infection, localized areas of tissue degeneration, or other complications. Although a small amount may be absorbed from the intestine when a large dose of insulin is protected from digestion, giving insulin orally is an expensive and erratic procedure, and many attempts have been made to find an oral insulin substitute. Within recent years, some success has been achieved.

As an outgrowth of early observations of hypoglycemia following sulfa-drug administration, the sulfonylureas have been found to be useful in controlling the blood sugar in many diabetics. It should be emphasized that they are not insulin substitutes, since they do not operate in the total absence of insulin, and are, therefore, ineffective in the depancreatized animal or the very severely diabetic human. It has been suggested that the compounds are effective by stimulating insulin output from the pancreas, or by some potentiation of what little insulin is secreted. There is some evidence for each of these proposed mechanisms, but the strongest support clearly favors stimulation of pancreatic β-cell secretion of insulin. One should remember the experiments cited earlier concerning exhaustion of overstimulated pancreatic islets. This must be a point of concern with long-term treatment of persons whose insulin-secreting mechanism is obviously inadequate although no widespread tendency toward complete β-cell failure has yet been noted clinically. Recent evidence also points to serious side effects with oral hyperglycemic agents such as Orinase.

HYPERGLYCEMIC AGENTS

Some time ago it was noted that a brief period of hyperglycemia preceded the usual fall in blood sugar produced by injection of insulin preparations from the United States, whereas many European preparations did not. Interest in the hyperglycemic glycogenolytic factor (HCF) led to the isolation from crude pancreas of a polypeptide consisting of 20 amino acids, which was distinct from insulin. The material produced a hyperglycemic response by releasing glucose by hydrolysis of glycogen from the liver. The pure polypeptide was renamed *glucagon*.

In animals treated with alloxan, in which the beta cells of the pancreatic islets are destroyed, diabetes develops readily; however, the hyperglycemic factor is still present in the pancreas even in the absence of insulin. Birds have islets rich in alpha cells, and they become hypoglycemic rather than hyperglycemic after pancreatectomy indicating a blood-sugar–regulating system dependent upon glucagon rather than insulin. On the other hand, treatment of an animal with cobalt salts results in a loss of the hyperglycemic factor from the pancreas with no apparent decrease in insulin production. This suggests that the site of production of the two materials is different. Histological examination of the alloxan-treated pancreas reveals destruction of the beta cells, while the alpha cells of the islets are injured by cobalt.

Glucagon is made in several tissues including the gastrointestinal tract and may be triggered in these sites by free amino acids and pancreazymin.

Further work has indicated that glucagon acts in the same manner as epinephrine and in fact is triggered by epinephrine during times of stress to accelerate phosphorylytic breakdown of glycogen, but only in the liver. In this organ, the resulting glucose-1-phosphate is rapidly changed to glucose-6-phosphate, which is split to glucose, leading to the observed hyperglycemia. Since it is devoid of actions on skeletal muscle metabolism or cardiovascular dynamics, glucagon is receiving attention in the management of hypoglycemia resulting from excess insulin. There is some evidence that glucagon exerts an additional catabolic action on protein metabolism.

The relationship between glucagon and insulin has been discussed. The control of this mechanism is diagramed in Figure 10.12. There

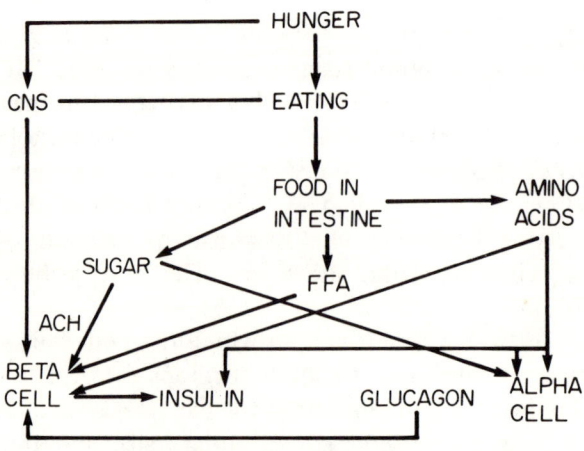

Figure 10.12. The reciprocal relationship between glucagon and insulin in the control of blood sugar indicating the trigger mechanisms.

is a complex relationship between insulin and glucagon because they respond in opposite directions to the same signal change in blood sugar. Exactly the same situation applies with respect to parathyroid hormone and calcitonin; however, it is probable that these are secreted continuously, whereas glucagon may be secreted only on demand.

Recently, a hormone has been isolated from the hypothalamus that specifically blocks the release of GH. The hormone *somatostatin* is synergistic with insulin. Alone, it will reduce blood sugar by permitting greater utilizations of glucose by somatic cells and improve insulin response. This fact, coupled with information that, in diabetes, insulin is deficient but glucagon is often present to excess, lead to further investigation of somatostatin. Somatostatin decreases *glucagon* levels as well as insulin, and it has been claimed that somatostatin will restore blood sugar concentrations to normal in the diabetic and alleviate other diabetic symptoms. Somatostatin has recently been found in the δ cells of the pancreatic islets. When released, it can *decrease* glucagon and insulin release simultaneously.

Somatostatin, an oligopeptide with 13 amino acids, can be easily synthesized. In fact, the search for active analogs is now under way.

Glucagon may have important consequences in diabetes. In diabetes, glucagon levels may be three times the normal level. In fasting, the glucagon level also changes. Normally, the glucagon-to-insulin secretion ratio is 0.3:1. In fasting, the ratio becomes 3:1. This may be a compensation to maintain the blood sugar until the brain can begin to utilize ketone, which requires some time.

DIABETES MELLITUS

This disease has already been identified as due to lack of insulin. In some instances, pancreatic β-cell function seems to be entirely missing, as judged from the lack of plasma insulin rise in response to Orinase. In many other cases, insulin is not only present, but the plasma level may be above normal, suggesting the involvement of other factors, such as somatotrophin, interfering with the normal sensitivity to insulin. Immunochemical assays have revealed many instances of elevated blood GH where plasma glucose is high.

Because of the short half-life of insulin, many methods have been tried to lengthen its span of action to avoid the need for treatment of diabetes by repeated injection. Several preparations have been devised that avoid this difficulty and decrease the rate of absorption from the injection site by using a combination of insulin with other substances to increase molecular size or even to yield an insulin suspension. At various times, histones, protamines, metals, and other materials have been used for this purpose. Such a depot insulin may be absorbed very slowly. A more satisfactory preparation is neutral protamine Hagedorn insulin (NPH), a combination of short-acting insulin to produce an immediate response together with a long-acting insoluble insulin to maintain the lowered blood sugar level for a longer time. Such a preparation is sometimes effective for longer than a day as compared to a few hours for the regular insulin preparation.

It has long been known that diabetes that commences at maturity may occur in the presence of a normal insulin-secretion rate. Such diabetes appears to be due to decreased insulin sensitivity. Several researchers, backed with experimental evidence, have suggested that diabetes may result from a deficiency of receptors and that the antidiabetic drugs act to increase binding of insulin to the cell by either increasing the number of receptors or increasing their sensitivity.

For these and other reasons, the recent treatment of diabetes has tended toward true replacement therapy to the extent of transplantation of pure beta cells into the organism.

Diabetes mellitus is a serious problem among Americans; approximately 3 of every 1,000 males and 5 of every 1,000 females in the United States have diabetes. The disease rate is increasing twice as fast as the increase in population. Although by no means an indictable relationship, carbohydrates now make up a higher proportion of the American diet than ever before, and the diabetic trend may represent a clinical counterpart to experimental depletion of the insulin-secreting mechanism. The incidence is conditioned by several factors:

1. *Sex*. About twice as many females as males have the disease.
2. *Age*. Diabetes increases in frequency with age, with a maxmum at 45 to 55 years. However, there is a distinct difference between the severe syndrome displayed by the juvenile diabetic and the more readily controlled disease in the middle-aged.

3. *Weight*. Obesity apparently increases the need of the body for insulin and depletes the islets, with resulting diabetes. In addition, the death rate for underweight diabetics is 36 percent less, and for overweight diabetics 57 percent greater, than the average weight population with diabetes. Weight loss is obviously an important procedure for overweight individuals.
4. *Heredity*. Diabetes is inherited as a recessive Mendelian trait. This may be the basis for the high incidence of the disease among Jews. Diabetes is less frequent among Orientals.
5. *Occupation*. The incidence of diabetes is greater in high-income groups, in city dwellers, and in persons who have sedentary occupations. This again may reflect the dietary difference contributing to obesity, although exercise itself has a beneficial effect upon metabolism in diabetics.

ENDOCRINE CONTROL OF ENERGY SOURCES

One of the most dramatic evidences of endocrine control is the mobilization of energy resources during exercise and starvation. In either case, massive alterations in supply and demand occur, and rates must be carefully adjusted to rapidly changing conditions.

The system for energy control is usually adjusted so that input and output of energy are balanced and the blood sugar changes around a set point of about 100 mgs%. The blood sugar control is not very accurate, and wide variations occur under normal conditions. The control system appears to be set so that there is no possibility of the blood sugar level dropping below about 60mgs% in order to preserve the integrity of the nervous system.

Under normal circumstances, the input-output balance is relatively constant. When the system is unfed for 24 or more hours, a series of events occur that more closely indicate the control that can be exerted. Within a short time (1 to 2 days), the blood sugar falls to a relatively constant value with very little variation and is maintained at this point for a long period of time (days). Figure 10.13 illustrates clearly the role of insulin and glucagon in mobilization of glucose and energy during various metabolic states and shows the competing activity of the two hormones in metabolic control. After a transient rise in level, glucagon falls and the level remains low, although teleol-

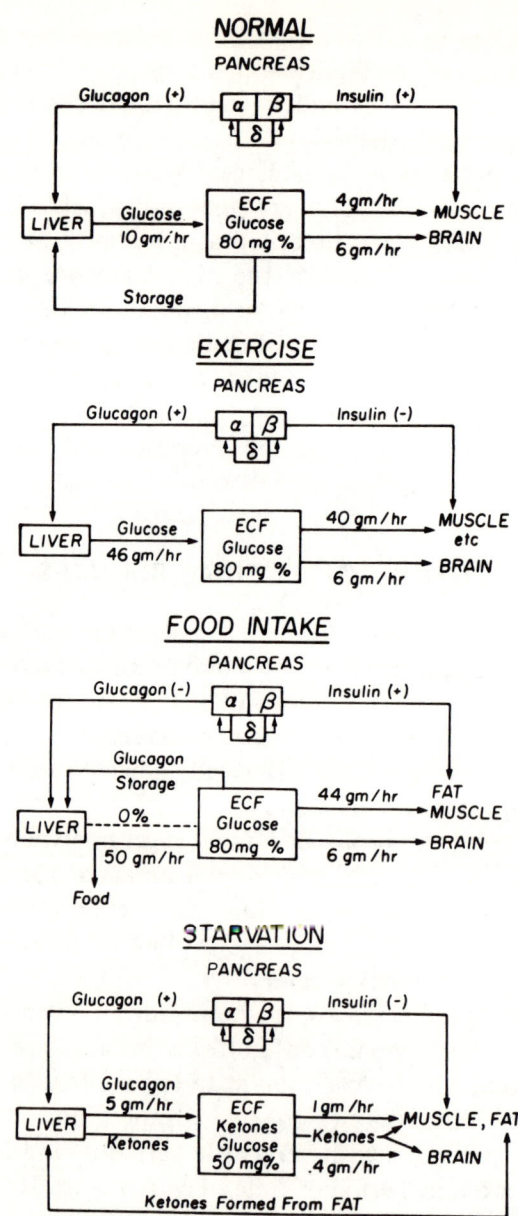

The Role of Insulin and Glucagon in Regulating Glucose to Maintain Blood Sugar. (Redrawn from Unger, R.H. Diabetic 25,136,1976)

Figure 10.13. Overall energy scheme for a fasting person.

ogy would indicate that it should rise to maintain the blood sugar. Insulin level falls, as would be expected.

General Metabolic Controls. In previous chapters, the interrelationships and coordination of metabolic functions have been discussed. The role of endocrine glands in the integration of the metabolic processes has been stressed. Nowhere is this coordination more evident than in the adaptive responses of an organism to starvation and exercise.

Chapter 8 (The Adrenal Medulla) clearly pointed out the coordinate role of the endocrines in mobilization of all possible energy sources for response to stress. The interaction of the medulla, the adrenal cortex, insulin and glucagon, STH, and other hormones occurs rapidly and smoothly.

An even greater coordination of resources is achieved by the body in starvation. A massive reorganization of energy resources occurs to conserve energy and release it only as necessary. Again, the endocrine organs play a vital role in the process.

The processes of control, which arise following the onset of starvation, occur in two phases: a short-term reaction followed by a long-term response. In the former, the blood sugar falls, which triggers the many mechanisms designed to restore blood glucose to normal levels, including release of epinephrine with consequent glycogenolysis and lipolysis; release of glucagon, which enhances glycogenolysis and lipolysis; suppression of insulin secretion, which decreases utilization and slows down anabolic processes; stimulation of the adrenal cortex with the resultant inhibition of utilization and stimulation of gluconeogenesis from the increased corticoid levels; and release of STH, which also effects peripheral glucose utilization.

If starvation continues, the glucose available for energy decreases from the lack of dietary intake and from decreasing internal supplies. The demands for energy sources continue. As a result, the body must turn to other mechanisms to maintain its integrity. Here again, a coordinated long-term effort is made. The glucose utilization of the tissues decreases to a minimum, and the cells actually become insulin-resistant. After a period of starvation, the response of the body to an increased insulin supply is much less than it is normally. The metabolic pathways that utilize glucose and the enzyme reactions that govern the rate appear to slow down. When a starved person is given a large dose of glucose, the glucose spills into the urine instead of being utilized by the cells to the same extent as in the nonstarved person.

The brain and muscle, which depend on glucose for energy, change their metabolic pattern. The brain, in particular, relies on glucose and does not need insulin to utilize it. After a period of starvation, the brain can begin to use ketone bodies, which are produced as a result of fat breakdown through processes discussed previously.

In the beginning of starvation, the metabolic processes stimulate a rapid breakdown of protein through the processes of gluconeogenesis to provide glucose. As starvation proceeds, these processes slow as does the breakdown of protein, although it never ceases. This may reflect a decrease in enzyme production, a reflection of the loss of most of the readily available protein, or a decreased responsiveness of the tissues. The liver assumes a new role in starvation. As protein is broken down, the liver and muscle rework the amino acids to conserve the essential amino acids and preferentially produce alanines and glutamines to be converted to energy sources. (See Figure 10.13.)

As starvation continues, the basal metabolic rate falls to about 50 percent of normal. This may reflect the conservation of resources, but the actual processes through which this occurs are not known. The adipocytes become insulin-resistant so that fat is conserved and less is broken down per unit time. The FFA acids that accumulate during starvation appear to directly inhibit utilization of glucose by cells. The number of insulin receptors in adipocytes can be correlated with size and number of fat cells, which may explain in part the changes in sensitivity that occur.

Other processes occur that help to govern the metabolic changes that take place in starvation. The balance between the glycogenolysis and gluconeogenesis is changed. When the glycogen stores are depleted, gluconeogenesis is stimulated to provide additional energy supplies. The level at which this occurs seems to be in the long-term activity of glucokinase.

There is also a feedback control between lipolysis and insulin. Elevation of ketone bodies in the blood as a result of lipolysis stimulates insulin production, which in turn inhibits lipolysis. There is another feedback because ketone bodies also directly inhibit lipolysis. The combination probably helps to conserve vital energy supplies. Many of these activities are shown in Figure 10.13, which clearly demonstrates the energy source flow and the utilization of energy in fasting.

Many of these processes may be reversed in the obese person. As fat is laid down over periods of time, the older fat cells become larger and more resistant to insulin. As mentioned, the number of receptors per cell decreases. Glucose tolerance is impaired, and insulin in the obese person has less effect. In fact, the obese person behaves very much like a diabetic in response to a glucose load. More calories are needed to maintain the obese person, and the intake must be correspondingly higher.

Exercise. In exercise, many of the same factors apply as in starvation but on a shorter time frame. Here again, energy output far surpasses input, and the body is forced to draw upon reserves. Once again, there is mobilization of glycogen stores followed by release of energy from fat and protein. The mechanisms are different. For the first few minutes of exercise, the blood sugar is maintained (1 hour), but after that time it begins to drop rapidly. The drop is paralleled by changes in both insulin and glucagon in the anticipated directions to maintain the blood sugar. The initial surge of glycogenolysis probably occurs because of the high epinephrine output triggered by the sudden demands of exercise.

In fact, the output of glucose from the liver more than doubles in the first hour, and 77 percent is derived from glycogen and about 23 percent from gluconeogensis. As exercise proceeds, the energy sources switch to FFA; at 240 minutes of exercise, 60 percent of the energy is derived from this source. The production of glucose is still relatively high (about 1.5 times normal), but the source has changed so that 50 percent is derived from lactate, 30 percent from glycerol, and 20 percent from amino acids.

The data obtained from starving or exercising subjects clearly indicate how energy can be mobilized on a high- or low-demand basis. It should also be emphasized that other endocrines contribute to the metabolic shifts. Corticoids are released and promote glyconeogensis. GH may be released under the changing blood sugar levels and contribute to the decreased sensitivity to insulin. Still other factors may be involved.

Mobilization of Energy Sources. One of the major components involved in mobilization of energy resources is the large store of energy in the fat cells of the body. The release of this energy occurs through many mechanisms. The FFA released are the ultimate source of energy. The FFA are normally bound to the albumin in plasma to the extent of 99.9 percent or more. Only the free FFA are active. (The effects of such binding on activity and of changes in concentration of blood protein can be reviewed in Chapter 6, The Thyroid.) Mechanisms of mobilization of FFA have been fiercely debated. For example, the decrease in insulin level during starvation may release the inhibition on release of FFA and inhibit synthesis of fat and thus raise the plasma level. Alternately, the release of catecholamines under the stress conditions of exercise or starvation may trigger FFA release.

Evidence originally indicated that FFA approximately doubled after a 48-hour fast and that norepinephrine had little effect on a further increase. The use of beta blockers to abort norepinephrine activity did prevent the rise in FFA. Nicotinic acid, which blocks cyclase activity but not the receptors, had no effect on FFA production. On the other hand, the use of theophylline, which prevents the phosphodiesterase breakdown of c-AMP, markedly stimulated FFA production. Fed and fasted animals had the *same maximum* rate of FFA production, indicating that starvation did *not increase* enzymatic activity. At 65 hours, the sensitivity of fat cells to norepinephrine disappears. However, when a beta blocker is used, the level of insulin also decreases. The addition of somatostatin, which blocks both insulin and glucagon secretion, had little effect on production of FFA at 65 hours of fasting.

We must conclude that norepinephrine has some effect in an early fast, but there is no explanation for mobilization of FFA in longer fasts. Known hormonal agents have little effect in longer fasts.

References

Anon. *Diabetes.* Kalamazoo, Michigan; Upjohn Co., 1960.
Berthet, J. "Some Aspects of the Glucagon Problem." *American Journal of Medicine* 26 (1959): 703.
Colwell, Q. R. "Tolbutamide Therapy after Five Years." *Diabetes 11 (Supplement)* 1 (1972).
Duncan, L. J. P. and J. D. Baird. "Compounds Administered Orally in Treatment of Diabetes Mellitus." *Pharm. Rev.* 12 (1960): 91.

Elbrink, J. and J. Bihler. *Membrane Transport Science.* **188** (1975): 1177.
Foa, P. P., G. Galansino, and G. Pozza. "Glucagon, a Second Pancreatic Hormone." *Recent Progr. Hormone Res.* **13** (1957): 473.
Fosham, P. H. "Current Trends in Research and Clinical Management of Diabetes." *Ann. N.Y. Acad. Sci.* **82** (1959): 195.
Knobil, E., and J. Hotchkiss. "Growth Hormone." *Ann. Rev. Physiol.* **26** (1964): 47.
Krahl, M. E. *Action of Insulin on Cells.* New York: Academic Press, 1961.
Lazarus, S. S. and B. W. Volk. *The Pancreas in Human and Experimental Diabetes.* New York: Gruen and Stratton, 1962.
Lefebre, P. J. and R. H. Unger. *Glucagon.* Oxford: Pergamon Press, 1972.
Levine, R., ed. "Symposium on Diabetes." *American Journal of Medicine* **31** (1961) 837.
Levine, R. and M. S. Goldstein. "Action of Insulin on Tissues, with some Remarks on Insulin Antagonism." *N.Y. State J. Med.* **62** (1962): 1236.
Manchester, K. L. and F. G. Young. "Insulin and Protein Metabolism." *Vit. Hormones* **19** (1961): 95.
Maugh, T. H. "Diabetes Therapy." *Science* **190** (1975): 1281.
———. "Insulin Receptors." *Science* **193** (1976): 220.
———. "New Hormonse Promise More Effective Therapy (Diabetes)." *Science* **188** (1975): 920.
Permutt, M. A. and D. M. Kipnis. "Insulin Biosynthesis and Secretion." *Fed. Proc.* **34** (1975): 1549.
Randle, P. J. "Endocrine Control of Metabolism." *Ann. Rev. Physiol.* **25** (1963): 291.
Randle, P. J. and H. E. Morgan. "Regulation of Glucose Uptake by Muscle." *Vit. Hormones* **20** (1962): 199.
Sharp, G. W., C. Wollhein, et al. "Studies on Mechanism of Insulin Release." *Fed. Proc.* **34** (1975): 1537.
Williams, R. H. *Diabetes.* New York: Paul B. Hoeber, 1960.
Winegrad, W. I. "Endocrine Effects on Adipose Tissue Metabolism." *Vit. Hormones* **20** (1962): 141.
Young, F. G., ed. "Insulin." *Brit. Med. Bull.* **16** (1960): 175.

11
Endocrinology of the Male

THE TESTES

The testis contains two major types of specialized tissues and the interstitial cells of Leydig. The tubules contain two types of cells: the *spermatogenic cells*, showing all forms of development from immature spermatogonia to mature spermatozoa, and the *Sertoli cells*, which are distinguished from the spermatogenic cells by structure and staining.

The most immature spermatogenic cells are close to the basement membranes, but, as maturation occurs through several stages of cell division, the maturing cells are pushed closer and closer to the lumen where the mature spermatozoa are released. The process of cell division and maturation occurs in two phases. The first phase, spermatocytogenesis, consists of mitotic division of a spermatogonium into a primary spermatocyte. As this spermatocyte is pushed away from the basement membranes toward the lumen, it matures and undergoes miotic division in which the 46 chromosomes originally present in the human are halved. Each of the new cells, now called *secondary spermatocytes*, contains either 22 + X chromosomes or 22 + Y chromosomes. The spermatocytes divide again to form the *spermatids*, which are said to be closely allied with the Sertoli cells and, in fact, appear to enter their cytoplasm. As they develop into mature sperm cells, they are squeezed off the Sertoli cells, and a new crop of spermatids enters. Therefore, the Sertoli cells are said to be *nutritional* in nature.

Special cells containing inclusion bodies are located in the connective tissue, fibroblasts, and blood vessels surrounding the tubules; these are the interstitial cells of Leydig, which are concerned with hormone production.

Function of the Testes. The testes perform several functions: they produce sperm, which are essential for reproduction; they are the principal source of androgens, which induce the secondary sexual characteristics of the male, including a definite psychological pattern; and they contain cells such as the Sertoli cells, which have characteristic supportive and metabolic functions, as discussed previously.

As with the female ovary, each testis is two organs in one: the tubules, which produce the sperm, and the interstitial cells, which appear to produce the male sex hormone, androgen. While it is possible to have normal androgen production in the absence of sperm production, the reverse is not possible since some androgen appears to be necessary to cause maturation of the sperm.

THE ANDROGENS

The male sex hormones are called *androgens*. They are C_{19}-steroids (Figure 11.1), with a hydroxyl or oxygen at positions 3 and 17. When an oxygen is present at C_{17}, the compounds are usually referred to as 17-ketosteroids. The two most common steroids to be isolated from the testes are *testosterone* and *androsterone*. Testosterone is presumed to be the steroid usually secreted by the cells of Leydig. If the urine of males is examined, many steroids of the 17-ketosteroid category can be found. These are probably steroids produced by the adrenal cortex as well as metabolic products of both testicular and adrenal hormones. When the testes of the male are removed, the excretion of 17-ketosteroids usually decreases about 40 percent.

Much of the information about the synthesis of the adrenocortical steroids can be carried over into the biological synthesis of the androgens. It is known that androgen can be synthesized in the body from both cholesterol and acetate. Progesterone is present in the testes

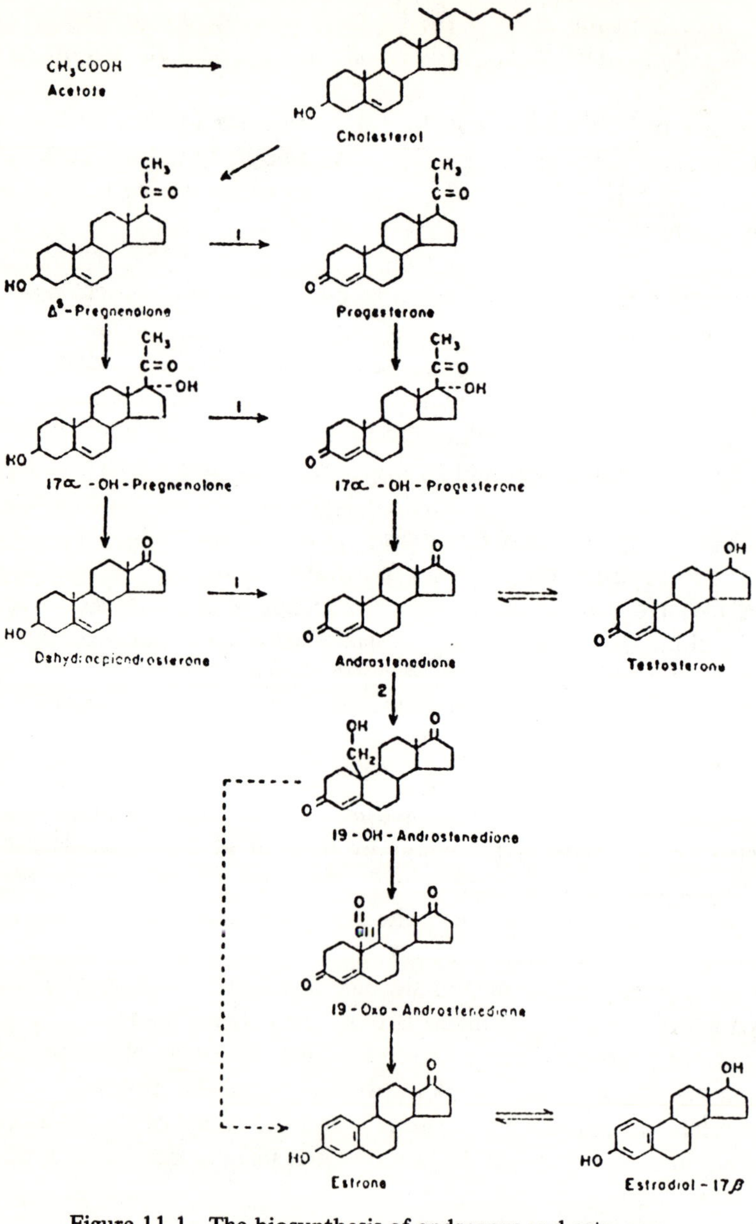

Figure 11.1. The biosynthesis of androgens and estrogens.

and indicates synthetic pathways similar to those of the adrenal cortex. Cyclic AMP is directly involved in synthesis when stimulated by ICSH. However, the action of the androgen itself on target tissue does not require c-AMP.

When androgens are administered to experimental animals or to patients, excretion of androgenic material including 17-ketosteroids in the urine is increased. Studies of the excretory products resulting from the administration of several androgens lead to the conclusion that testosterone is converted in part to androsterone, which is excreted in the urine. It has also been well documented that testosterone can be converted to estrogen in the testis. A large part of the androgen is metabolized by the liver and excreted by the kidney with a considerable portion being excreted in the bile.

If the activities of the steroids are compared, it is found that testosterone is about two to four times as active as androsterone. Absolute comparisons are not satisfactory since the method of assay produces different evaluations of relative activities. Alteration in the molecular structure also produces variations in relative activity. Synthetic addition of a benzoate molecule to testosterone, for example, will increase the activity about 10 times, presumably because of prolonged absorption.

Many assays are available for the determination of androgens in blood and urine. One of the most common measures the amount of 17-ketosteroids. This method gives consistent values at normal steroid levels and can be used to detect changes in testicular function, but is only an indirect measure, since testosterone, the major androgen secreted by the testis, is not a 17-ketosteroid. Since most of the androgens present in both blood and urine are conjugated with sulfate and, to a lesser degree with glucuronide, it is usually necessary to hydrolyze the sample with mineral acid before extracting with an organic solvent in order to obtain the free steroids, which are artifacts of the method and do not occur in nature.

The most common biological assay is probably the increased weight response of the ventral prostate of the rat to injected androgen. The seminal vesicle weight response and the increase in size of the capon comb are among many other suggested methods for androgen assay. Any bioassay of mixtures of substances with such widely differing biological activities must be approached with caution.

THE ANDROGENS AS SEX HORMONES

The functioning of the androgens as sex hormones is most clearly shown by the characteristic changes in the male at puberty. As androgen production begins, the testes begin to grow, followed by growth of the penis and of axillary and pubic hair. The hair regresses to the male hairline, and the beard develops. The voice deepens, the sweat glands develop, and the breasts may enlarge from estrogen production. Increased muscle protein is laid down, and weight and height may increase dramatically. The excretion of gonadotrophins may be rather low, but the 17-ketosteroids in the urine increase steadily in the male until they reach adult levels, at about 18 years of age.

In the prepubertal castrate, these changes do not occur. If castration occurs postpubertally, many of the sex characteristics regress. In the individual castrated before puberty, there is a disproportionate growth of long bones, and the height may be much above normal. In the female given androgens (or in whom adrenal tumor develops), typically male sex characteristics may be produced, such as deep voice, beard, baldness, redistribution of body fat and protein, and failure of menstruation, and the breasts may atrophy.

Along with the physical developments of puberty, many psychic changes occur in the male. The sex drive begins, together with the ability to perform the sex act. Androgen influences the erectile tissue of the penis, but erections can be obtained in infants. Contrary to much popular opinion, the castrate is able to produce an erection and to perform the sex act, probably through retention of conditioning, if it was learned previous to castration. Since a great part of the emission fluid of ejaculation is formed by glands of the seminal vesicles and the prostate, which are maintained by androgen, castration decreases the ability to ejaculate although it may not be abolished, even in the face of decreased formation of seminal fluid. Androgen receptors have been closely identified in many of the secondary sex organs. The receptors are decreased by hypophysectomy and are increased by FSH (but not by any other pituitary hormone).

From the foregoing, it is apparent that two types of hypofunction can occur in the male genital system: decreased androgen secretion and failure to produce sperm. Either one may lead to a common problem demanding clinical attention, *infertility*, which is not always synonymous with *sterility*. Recently, a new approach to this problem has been to administer large doses of androgen, which depresses sperm formation and its release from the tubules. When the androgen is withdrawn after such treatment, a *rebound phenomenon* occurs, in which the sperm count may rise to levels much above normal for the particular individual. Some success has been reported with this method.

The function of the gonads in the female usually ceases in the fourth or fifth decade. In men, the function may continue into old age. However, in some men there is reported to be a testicular failure, which occurs about 10 years later than the female menopause. This period, the *male climacteric*, has many symptoms of the female menopause. When this condition is due solely to failure of androgen production, replacement therapy is very satisfactory. More often, psychic factors are so strongly involved that testosterone alone does not solve the problems.

Control of Hormone Secretion. The mechanisms that induce androgen secretion by the testes are not well understood. Although little or no androgen can be detected in the urine of young children or animals, it has been reported that hypophysectomy at birth will lead to typical regression changes in the accessory sex organs. Furthermore, relatively large amounts of gonadotrophin are present in the pituitaries of young males. Again, the young male child can respond to the injection of gonadotrophin long before the usual onset of puberty. Puberty, the time of developing sexual maturity, occurs in males at about 12 to 16 years of age, resulting in full sex characteristics at about 18 years of age. There is no indication of the mechanism that triggers the onset of puberty, the release of gonadotrophin, and the secretion of the sex hormones. Certain brain lesions will cause premature onset of puberty, and, from this meager evidence, it has been said that the hypothalamus causes the release of gonadotrophin at the proper time. However, this does not answer the question, since there is no indication of why the proper time occurs at this particular age. It has been well demonstrated in rats that at puberty the accessory sex glands (seminal vesicles, prostate, etc.) respond to much lower doses of androgen than at any time earlier or later in life. Although this may explain why low doses of androgen are effective, it does not explain why the tissues suddenly become more sensitive at the particular time denoted at puberty.

The control of androgen secretion is vested in the pituitary (Figure

11.2) as mediated by hypothalamic influences. There is a feedback system between ICSH (interstitial cell stimulating hormone, identical to LH) and the production of testosterone by the testes. Administration of ICSH results in increased steroid excretion and the development of secondary sex characteristics, even in the immature animal.

Sperm production is under the control of FSH; in tubule deficiencies, the output of FSH is high regardless of androgen output and development of normal sex characteristics. The feedback system for FSH has not been isolated, but must exist, since the normal individual has sperm production and low FSH output. The testes cannot produce sperm in the absence of androgen, but it can produce androgen in the absence of sperm.

Although testosterone is the primary androgen produced by the testes and apparently serves as the feedback to higher centers, evidence suggests that it must be converted to dihydrotestosterone (DHT) before it becomes active at the tissue levels. The tissue receptors appear to bind DHT more effectively than testosterone, and only DHT is preferentially retained by the nuclei of target cells. In certain tumors, only DHT is active. DHT may be more effective than testosterone for these reasons in much the same way as triiodothyronine is more active than thyroxine.

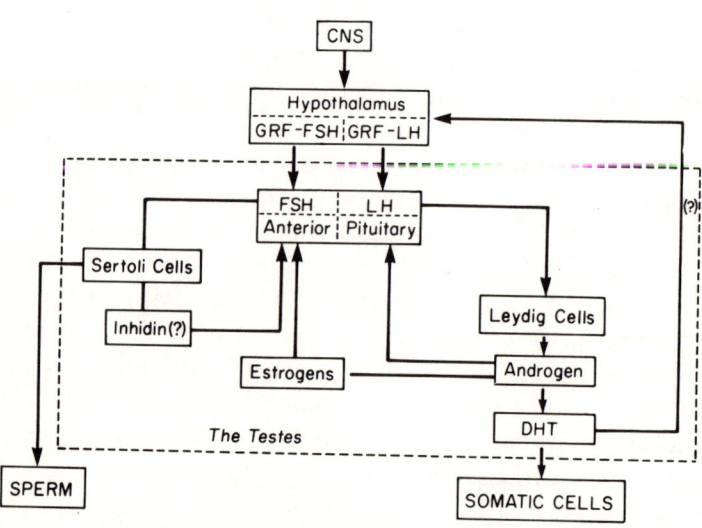

Figure 11.2. The control system of the testes indicating two systems, one for androgen production and one for sperm production.

Androstendione and testosterone, which may occur in large amounts, are also precursors of estrogen synthesis in the testes. In fact, stallions are used for commercial production of estrogen.

One of the more interesting aspects of androgen activity is its effect on the hypothalamus. Some evidence exists that DHT is produced in the hypothalamus and that the extent of production is under feedback control of testosterone. This could mean that the higher centers are influenced directly by metabolites. An interesting aspect of the feedback mechanism is the oscillation in LH concentration at regular intervals of 2 to 3 hours in the male, for totally unknown reasons.

Two methods of control have been postulated. McCullagh proposed that a hormone "inhibin" was produced from the spermatogenic tubules, and that this hormone acts to suppress FSH secretion during normal sperm production. A water-soluble testis extract was reported to have suppressed FSH production in castrated males. Other researchers believe that the evidence is stronger that estrogen produced by the testes is the specific FSH inhibitor, and it is true that, in the stallion, extremely large quantities of estrogen are produced by the testes. The Sertoli cells are assumed to be the site of estrogen production. However, in certain clinical entities such as Klinefelter's syndrome, where the tubules are missing or nonfunctional and Leydig cells are present, the individual secretes rather large quantities of estrogen, presumably because of the high gonadotrophin titer that results from lack of feedback. In this situation, FSH production apparently stimulates estrogen production and the latter does not inhibit FSH production. This indicates either that some other inhibitor must be present or that specific receptors are absent.

In Klinefelter's disease, the male may develop a bizzare set of conditions in which the testes are small and do not produce sperm despite an apparently normal male developmental pattern. The excretion of 17-ketosteroids is normal or slightly low, but the excretion of FSH may be high. Some of these patients have a female Barr chromatin pattern because of the presence of at least two X (female sex) chromosomes, together with one Y (male sex) chromosome, whereas the normal male human has the unpaired X and Y combination. Thus, these patients are genetically female, while their phenotype is typically male. Abnormal chromatin distributions are found in both male and female. In the female, the condition is usually associated with ovarian dysgenesis.

In the hypophysectomized rat, FSH restores and maintains spermatogenesis without affecting secondary sex characteristics, while LH will independently maintain sex characteristics and steroid excretion. Spermatogenesis cannot be maintained indefinitely without some androgen. When the testes are removed, the basophils of the pituitary develop large vacuoles and other characteristic changes, known collectively under the term *castration cells*, and the gland liberates large quantities of gonadotrophin, mostly FSH. The appearance of the pituitary and its hormone content can be reversed by administration of androgen. Large amounts of androgen will prevent synthesis of gonadotrophin by the pituitary and suppress spermatogenesis, resulting in testicular atrophy. Furthermore, for reasons not well understood, the administration of androgen to hypophysectomized animals immediately after operation will maintain spermatogenesis, but if the degeneration of the testes is allowed to occur before treatment is started, androgen has no effect.

INTERRELATIONS BETWEEN THE TESTES AND OTHER ORGAN SYSTEMS

There is a close relation between the testes and other endocrine organs. Castration is followed by some atrophy of the thyroid, and administration of testosterone results in thyroid hypertrophy. Removal of the thyroid affects sexual function and, to some extent, the production of sperm. This may be due to the generally low metabolic rate in the thyroidectomized animal, rather than a specific effect. The relationship of the testis to the adrenal is also well documented. The female adrenal is larger than that of the male, and the administration of androgen will reduce it in size. In the mouse, an inner zone of the cortex, the *X-zone*, is present at birth and remains in the male until androgen production occurs, when it regresses. In the female, it persists until androgens are administered or until the animal becomes pregnant, when the increased androgen production by the placenta and adrenals causes regression. The human adrenal also has a so-called fetal-zone, or X-zone, which regresses after birth. Adminstration of androgen has been reported to decrease adrenocortical steroid output; in young rats, male sexual function can be maintained by adrenal androgens, showing the close relationship between the two organs. The menopausal female often develops masculizing traits because estrogens are no longer being produced, but the adrenal continues to produce about 12 milligrams per day of 17-ketosteroids, which are free to produce androgenic effects.

Extrasexual Activity of Androgens. Besides their activity as sex hormone, the androgens have a generalized effect on the body. The administration of androgen to both animals and human beings results in a definite nitrogen retention not seen with other hormones. This nitrogen retention has been demonstrated even during catabolism of protein in patients in fasting states. In general, the nitrogen-retaining ability of the physiological steroids is correlated with androgenicity, but synthetic steroids have been produced in which this is not the case. Perhaps as a result of the nitrogen retention or of a specific growth factor, androgens cause marked growth of both liver and kidney. Protein retention also leads to formation of the bony matrix followed by calcium and phosphorus deposition. This effect has been used clinically in treating osteoporosis. The androgens share a salt- and water-retaining action with both estrogens and adrenocortical steroids. Androgens probably have some influence on fat metabolism, considering the difference in distribution and amount of fat between male and female, although it is difficult to precisely differentiate the androgen from a positive estrogen effect.

Particular interest has been aroused in certain derivatives of the sex hormones, especially derivatives of testosterone. By a proper selection of substituent groups, it is first possible to separate the activities of the molecule so that the effect on nitrogen metabolism (myotrophic activity) can be separated from the androgenicity. Second, some compounds with progestational effects are potent pituitary gonadotrophin inhibitors and are being used for fertility control in the female. Finally, some of the compounds have been demonstrated to have a very interesting action in stimulating sperm production in cases of infertility. Many compounds have been devised with varying properties. The side-chain and the other substitutions on the C_{17} atom in the androgen molecule may be a variety of groups, chosen to produce the desired degree of androgenic, progestational, or myotrophic effect.

References

Burrows, H. *Biological Actions of Sex Hormones.* New York: Cambridge University Press, 1949.

Bishop, W. et al. "Acute and Chronic Effects of Hypothalamic Lesions on Release of FSH, LH and LTH," *Endoc.* 91 (1972): 673.

Dorfman, R. I., and R. A. Shipley. *Androgens.* New York: John Wiley & Sons, 1956.

Greep, R. O. *Reproductive Physiology.* Baltimore: University Park Press, 1974.

———. "Male Reproductive System." *Handbook of Physiology.* Bethesda, Maryland: Amer. Physiol. Soc., 1975.

Nelson, W. O. and J. Macleod. "Biology of the Testes." *Ann. N.Y. Acad. Sciences* 55 (1952): 545.

Young, W. C. *Sex Internal Secretions.* 2 vols. Baltimore: Williams & Wilkins, 1961.

12
Endocrinology of the Female

THE OVARY

The ovary is the reproductive organ of the female. Two distinct types of cells begin to develop in the analags: large cells, which will become the germinal cells or *ova*, grow and become separated by smaller cells, which will eventually become the *granulosa*. The granulosa cells gradually surround each primordial ovum and form the beginning of a follicle. There are follicles in a rudimentary state in the fetal ovary but they do not develop further until puberty. The cortex contains many thousands of follicles, which decrease in number as the years of sexual activity continue.

The Ovarian Follicle. Histologically, there are several types of follicles. The primary follicles are the immature state in which most follicles exist. They are concentrated in the periphery of the cortex of the ovary and consist of a large egg cell surrounded by a layer of granulosa cells. In the second stage, the follicles become growing organs, as distinguished from the quiescent cells just mentioned. The growth is largely in the follicular cells or granulosa, but also involves the enclosed ovum. As the follicle grows, the ovum develops to one side, and follicular cells are broken down to produce fluid which fills a central cavity, the *antrum*. As development reaches a later stage, the mature follicle consists of an ovum (the largest cell in the body), surrounded by granulosa cells, a large fluid-filled cavity surrounded by a thin layer of follicular cells, and an outer membrane (Figure 12.1).

A single cell of the germinal epithelium may give rise to many primary ova. Once the follicle is formed, each primary ovum (or *oocyte*) can give rise to only one mature germ cell. Before expulsion of the germ cell at ovulation, the cell divides several times, expelling so-called polar bodies and reducing the number of chromosomes to 23 instead of the 46 normally present in the other cells of the body. The original number of chromosomes is restored by a combination of male and female germ cells. In the human, all normal ova contain $22 + X$ chromosomes. The sperm are sex-determining, since addition of $22 + X$ to the ova will yield $44 + XX$ (female genotype) and $22 + Y$ will yield $44 + XY$ (male genotype). As already discussed in Chapter 11, genotypic abnormalities will result from combinations such as $44 + XO$ (Turner's syndrome) or $44 + XXY$ and $44 + XXXY$ (Klinefelter's syndrome).

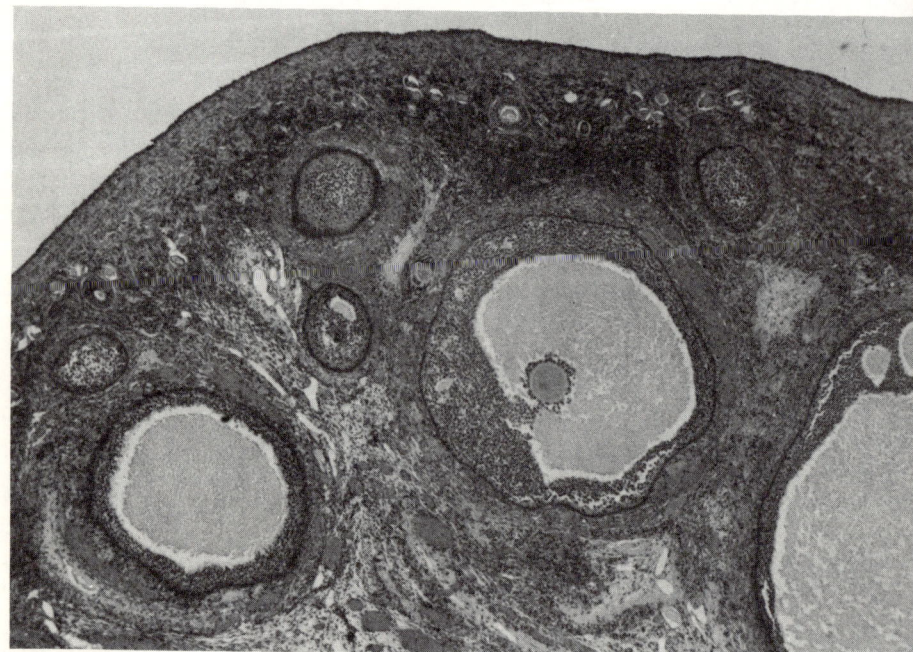

Figure 12.1. The follicular development in the ovary.

Since Lipner has shown no increase in intrafollicular tension with continued growth of the follicle, enzymatic rupture of the follicle must take place, resulting in the escape of both fluid and ovum. If rupture does not occur for some reason, the follicle regresses and becomes cystic. Following escape of the ovum, the alteration in hormonal and physical factors causes a rapid growth of the remaining granulosa cells, which develop into a new hormone-secreting organ, the corpus luteum. Unless pregnancy intervenes, the corpus luteum soon begins to regress, the yellow color disappears, and an inactive *corpus albicans* is formed.

Since the ovary was known to secrete two distinct types of endocrine substances, estrogens and progesterone, there was long a tendency to associate these with the maturing follicle and the corpus luteum, respectively, which are both under the control of the anterior pituitary. The present evidence is that the *theca interna* of the ovary produces most, if not all, of the estrogen, much as the interstitial cells of the testis produce testosterone. The granulosa was implicated for many years, but experiments in which the granulosa was destroyed by X ray without markedly affecting the production of estrogen failed to sustain its role as an endocrine organ. No progesterone is secreted by the follicle until the luteal cells are formed after ovulation. On the other hand, estrogen secretion continues after the formation of the corpus luteum, indicating a separate source for the two major female hormones.

THE FEMALE SEX HORMONES

The Estrogens and Progesterone. It is probable that the ovary secretes 17-beta estradiol as the physiological estrogen (Figure 12.2). The two other estrogens that occur in the blood and urine—*estrone* and *estriol*—are believed to be metabolites of estradiol, as demonstrated by experiments in which each of the hormones is given to a female mammal and all three forms are isolated. If estriol is given, only estriol can be located. If estrone is given, both estrone and estriol and a little estradiol can be found, while, if estradiol is administered, all three hormones can be isolated, indicating the metabolic sequence. The outstanding chemical structure in estrogens is the phenolic character of the A-ring, which readily permits separation from 17-ketosteroids and adrenocortical steroids and provides

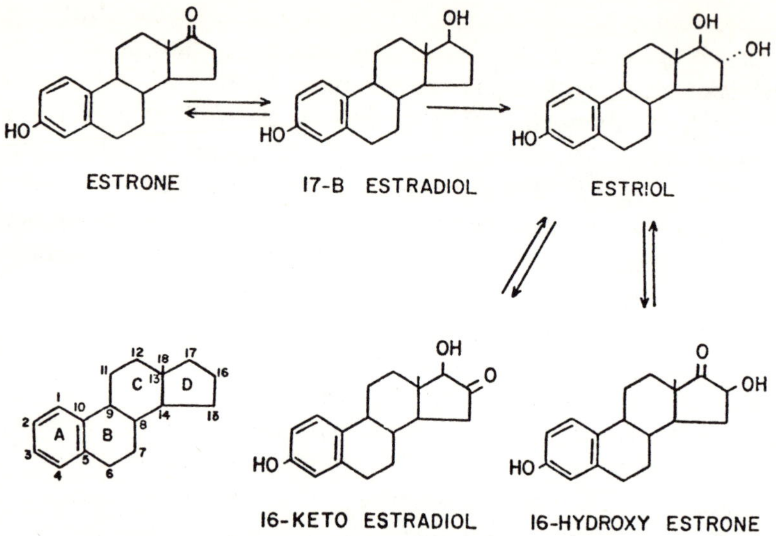

Figure 12.2. The estrogens and their metabolic scheme.

a means of positive chemical identification and semiquantitative estimation.

The biological activity of the estrogens to some extent follows the pattern of metabolism; estradiol is by far the most potent, with estriol and estrone following, in that order. Both relative and absolute potencies show wide variations, depending upon the tests employed. For example, similar vaginal cytological responses are produced by dosage ratios of 1:3:12 for estradiol:estriol:estrone. For uterine-weight responses, the same steroids have a ratio of 1:5:20; for vaginal opening, the ratios are about 1:20:30. This again illustrates the fallibility of biological assay.

The estrogens appear to be formed from cholesterol by processes similar to those leading to the synthesis of the adrenal corticoids (Figure 12.2). However, the estrogens that are isolated following administration of C^{14}-labeled acetate do not have C^{14} in the phenolic A-ring, which suggests that this is not synthesized by the acetate pathway. In comparison to the output of steroid by the adrenal cortex and the testes, the ovary produces very small quantities of estrogen. It is probable that only a few micrograms per day are produced and liberated into the bloodstream (Table 12.1). A portion of the estrogen in the blood probably exists as free steroid,

Table 12.1. Relationships among the principal estrogens in the human female in terms of excretion and biological activity.

Estrogen	Spontaneous Excretion (μg/day)	Relative Activity (Uterine Weight Test)
Estradiol	2-19	100
Estriol	6-27	15
Estrone	5-20	5

but considerable quantities are found as conjugates with sulfuric and glucuronic acids. Perhaps 50 percent or more of the circulating estrogen is also bound to plasma proteins of the α-globulin type. Estrogen may also circulate in the bloodstream in the form of *pro-estrogen*, an inactive form, which is converted into an active form at tissue sites. The liver has been suggested as one of the major sites of this conversion.

Inactivation of estrogen occurs very rapidly in the living animal. Enzymatic activity in the liver results in both destruction of the estrogen molecules and conversion to less active steroids. The degraded estrogen is partially excreted in the urine and partially in the bile. Removal or damage of the liver results in continued stimulation of accessory sex organs from circulating estrogens, which would normally be destroyed. Impairment of estrogen inactivation, which occurs in protein- and vitamin-deficiency states, may be a reflection of a generally decreased liver function, rather than of any specific alteration in degradative pathways.

Assay of the ovarian hormones has always been difficult. The extremely small quantities of hormone present and the lack of suitable chemical or biological methods for estimation of the hormones in blood have complicated the picture. A convenient biological assay is the response of the uterus of the rat or mouse to injected estrogen. Since estrogen causes salt and water retention by the uterus, a simple assay based upon increase in weight following injection of the desired material is provided. The major difficulty is the high degree of variability. The estrogens can also be determined photochemically by their fluorescence under ultraviolet light after treatment with strong acid (Kober method). Chemical methods are available for the determination of progesterone and its metabolites, but none of them is very specific or very sensitive.

Biological methods for progesterone assay are poor and are based primarily upon measurements of *deciduomata* formed in rat uteri, or development of a secretory endometrium in various animals primed with estrogen.

Influence of Estrogens on Metabolic Processes. Estrogens exert a metabolic effect far beyond that directly concerned with the genitalia. Large doses of estrogens have an anabolic effect on the metabolism of protein and act to decrease the utilization of carbohydrate. The administration of estrogen may produce diabetes in the rat after a sensitivity has been created by partial pancreatectomy and a high carbohydrate diet. The estrogens may also affect the metabolism of fats and carbohydrates.

Mammalian females have a greater tendency to develop ketosis on fasting than do males, suggesting some influence of estrogens on fat catabolism. In birds, the administration of estrogen results in hyperlipemia and hypercholesterolemia, in contrast to the well-known lower incidence of these changes in the human female. Estrogens also affect the retention of salt and water in the tissue, which may explain the occurrence of edema during the estrogenic phase of the menstrual cycle. The female sex hormone influences the maintenance of a positive calcium balance, and, in persons with an estrogen deficiency, decalcification of the long bones occurs, which can be restored by administration of the hormone.

Control of Ovarian Function. The ovary in many ways behaves as if it were two separate endocrine systems. On one hand, the production of FSH by the pituitary triggers the production of estrogen by the ovarian thecal cells. The estrogen then serves to complete the feedback loop. On the other hand, the production of progesterone that occurs in the corpus luteum is stimulated by LH, and progesterone is the feedback control. Unfortunately, the situation is not clear-cut because some LH may be required to produce estrogen, and some estrogen may be required to produce progesterone and to complete the progesterone feedback loop. In addition, LTH maintains the corpora lutea in many species and apparently is part of the progesterone feedback loop. Much of the feedback may be at the hypothalamic level, and the interactions may also be at this point (Figure 12.3).

ENDOCRINOLOGY OF THE FEMALE 203

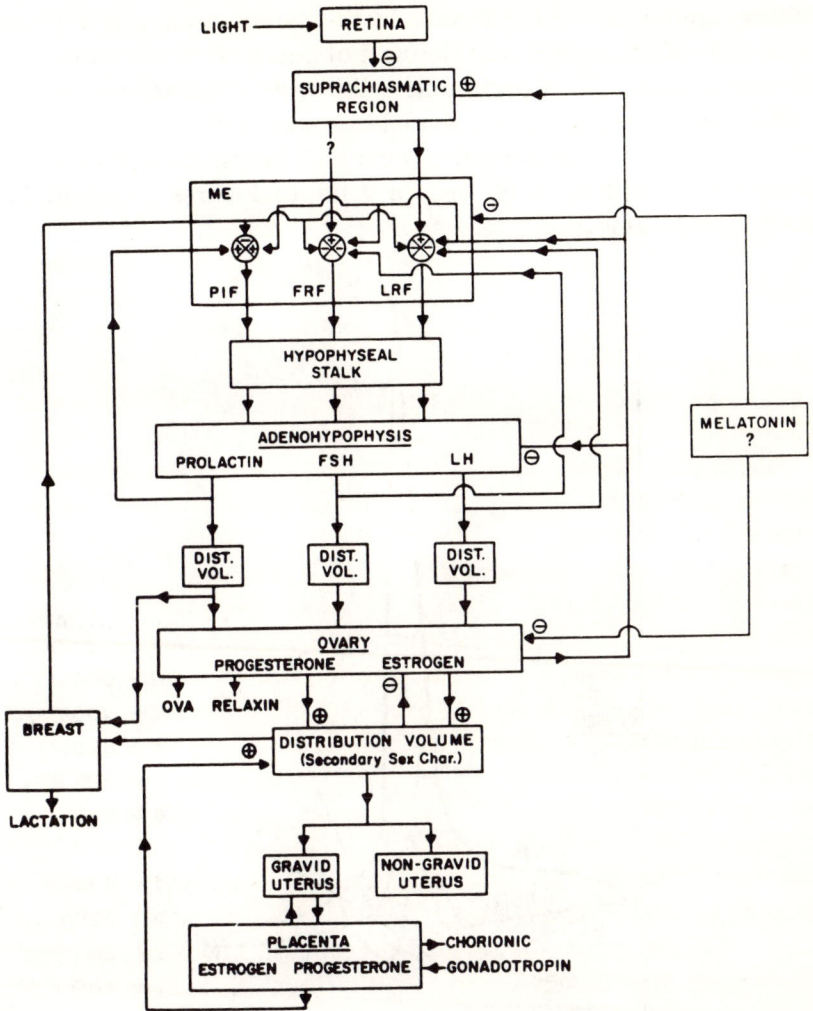

Figure 12.3. The control system for gonatrophin secretion. (With permission from Stear and Kadish, *Hormone Control Systems*, Amer. Elsevier, New York, 1976.)

The control system, however, is not a total summary of ovarian activity. The most striking phenomena are the menstrual cycle and pregnancy. Beginning at about age 12 and continuing until about age 45, the average woman has 28-day cycles. These cycles represent the growth of a follicle, maturation of the ovum, rupture of the follicle, conversion of the follicle to the corpus luteum, and, finally, regression of the follicle and the start of a new cycle. Because of the hormonal changes that occur during the cycle, there are also periodic fluctuations in the secondary sexual characteristics.

To understand the control system and its resultant physiological responses, it will be necessary to refer to Figures 12.4 and 12.5 during the ensuing discussion.

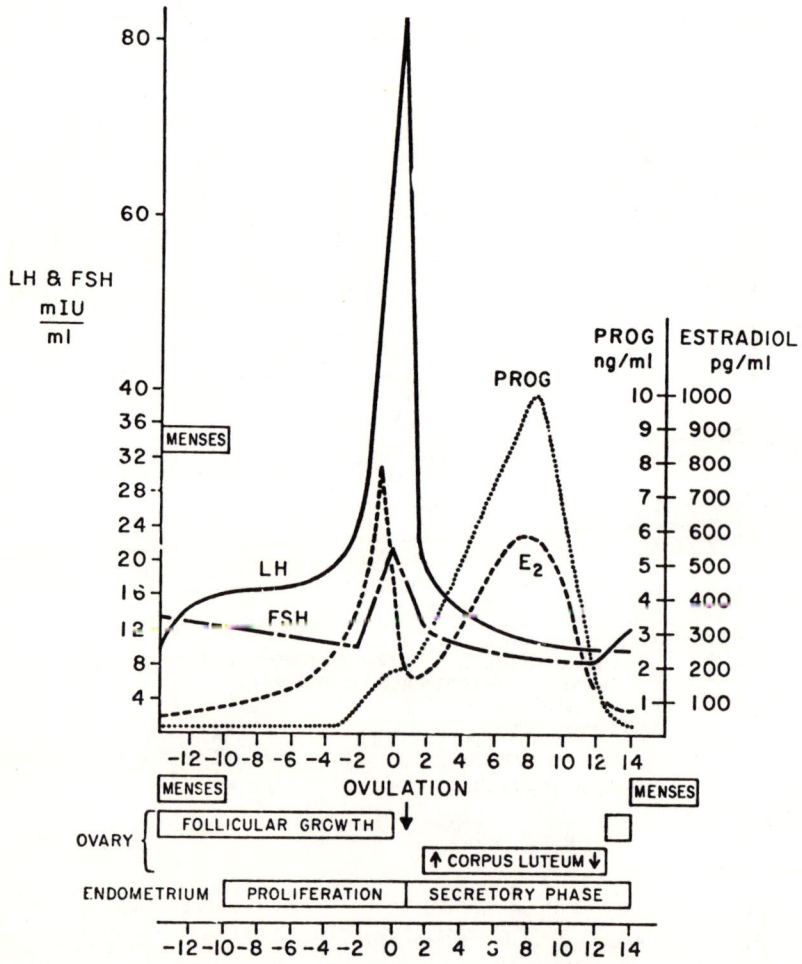

Figure 12.4. The physical events and changes in the endocrine secretions during the course of a normal menstrual cycle, including the estrogens, progesterone, pituitary hormones, and the uterus.

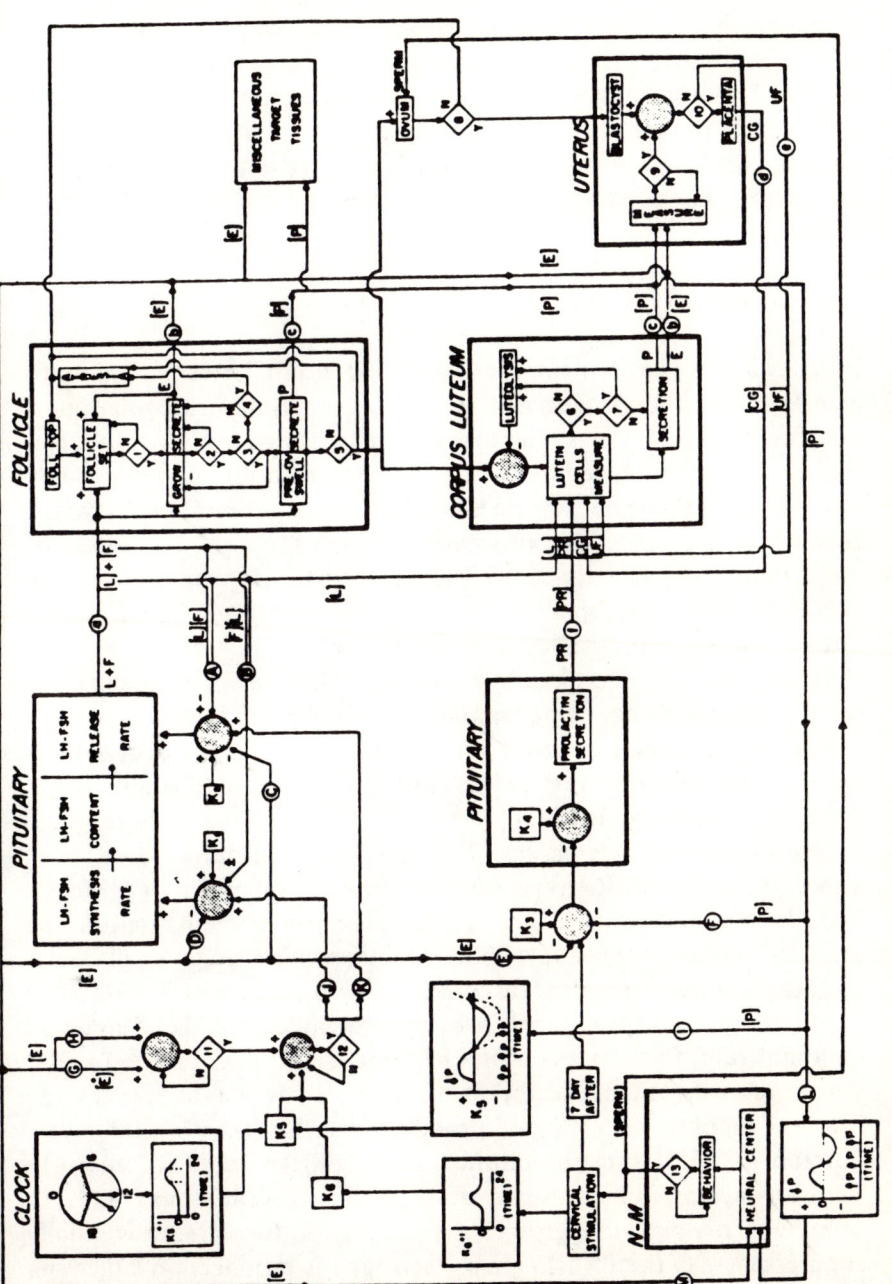

Figure 12.5. The biological clock governing the sexual cycle in rats and the control of the events within it. (Taken from Brown and Gann, *Engineering Principles in Physiology*, Academic Press, 1975.)

It has already been mentioned (Chapter 3) that there are many circadian rhythms in bodily processes. In fact, the menstrual cycle is one of the most well known and most constant. The exact trigger for the biological clock is not known. The onset of menstruation (*menarche*) occurs for no known reason. Various suppositions regarding sensitivity of receptors, sudden increase in hormone levels, and so on, have been proposed, but these do not answer the basic question.

THE MENSTRUAL CYCLE

It has already been mentioned that the normal female begins to menstruate at puberty and that the process continues at regular intervals for about 35 years, ceasing with menopause. Menstruation is the cyclic uterine bleeding, which occurs at approximately 28-day intervals in the normal female and involves many hormonal, psychic, and other factors. The processes occurring before the onset of menstruation in each cycle are preparatory for implantation, vascularization, and development of the fertilized ovum. Menstruation intervenes only if pregnancy does not occur.

It is unfortunate that much work on cyclic behavior has been done on the rat, which does *not* parallel cyclic behavior in primates. The following discussion is based on primate physiology. Correlations between the species must be carefully evaluated before any correspondence can be accepted.

The menstrual cycle may be described in general terms. Following a menstrual period, the reproductive system is quiescent. (Although logically the cycle should start at the cessation of menstruation, the practical difficulty of determining exactly when this takes place has dictated the usual practice of commencing a cycle with the onset of menstruation.) The uterus has been denuded of the functional endometrium, the corpus luteum has regressed, a new follicle has not yet developed, and the secretion of hormones is at a low level. The lowered amount of estrogen produced by the ovary initiates production of FSH from the pituitary, and follicles begin to grow. In the human, one follicle usually grows faster than the others, and, for unknown reasons, the growth of all except the largest is finally suppressed. As the follicle grows, estrogen is produced in larger and larger amounts; some evidence indicates that small amounts of LH may be necessary to cause estrogen production. The increased estrogen titer produces a rapid growth of the endometrium, with development of increased arterial blood supply and glands. This is the uterine proliferative phase. At the same time, the cells of the vagina become cornified. The production of estrogen decreases FSH output by the pituitary, and LH release is stimulated either by the increased estrogen or the decreased FSH concentration.

At some optimal concentration of FSH and LH, perhaps combined with structural weakness with increasing size, the growing follicle is enlarged to the point of rupture. The released ovum is transported to the fallopian tubes and thence to the uterus for fertilization. Granulosa cells in the ruptured follicle now begin to proliferate and form lutein cells. In the rat, LH initiates formation of the corpus luteum but does not cause it to secrete. In fact, small amounts of progesterone will prevent the LH rise and subsequent events. The release of LH is cyclic, being released at 1 to 2-hour intervals in the preluteal phase and at 4-hour intervals during the luteal phase. The shift apparently occurs under the influence of estrogen. In the rat, it is probable that secretion is induced by luteotrophin (LTH, identical with prolactin) release from the pituitary or by rising LH titer, and progesterone is formed in large amounts under LTH stimulation. Precise information on mechanisms leading to release of LTH is lacking, as it also is on trophic processes resulting in progesterone secretion in species such as the human, which may be lacking LTH.

Progesterone prepares the endometrium for pregnancy by inducing growth of the cells, water retention, greater vascularity, and glandular development (the secretory phase). The vaginal cells become less cornified and develop into a squamous epithelium. The rising concentration of progesterone now suppresses the production by the pituitary of LH and possibly LTH, which, in turn, decreases progesterone production; such inhibition may require the presence of estrogen.

It has also been mentioned that the prostaglandins may inhibit LTH and thus bring about the fall in progesterone production; in fact, a peak of prostaglandin production occurs in the ovary just as the steroid levels begin to decrease. Luteolysis occurs only in the presence of the uterus, which secretes PGF (prostaglandin F). If pregnancy intervenes, the corpus luteum secretion is maintained at a high rate for some time by placental hormones. In the absence of pregnancy, progesterone production declines. The endometrium, which has been maintained in a turgid condition by the salt and water retention, decreases in thickness; the arteries are compressed; and, in consequence, the blood supply is decreased. At this time, there is also a decreased production of estrogen, which decreases the blood supply. This leads to necrosis of the endometrium and sloughing-off of the dead cells. It has been suggested that this process is further enhanced by a menstrual *toxin*, which increases fragility of the blood vessels.

The entire process of menstruation is under the control of a *biological clock*. Schwartz has worked out a feedback model, which takes into consideration most of the known facts about the cyclic behavior (Figure 12.5).

During menstruation, there is a discharge from the uterus consisting of cells, mucus, and blood, but no obvious clotting of the menstrual fluid. Since a fibrinolytic enzyme is present in the detritus, some authorities now claim that the blood does clot initially but is liquefied again before discharge. As a result of the sloughing process, the endometrium is denuded to the *basalis*. The corpus luteum continues to decrease in activity and regresses in size. There is now an increase in FSH titer stimulated by the low estrogen levels with the growth of a new follicle, and the entire process is repeated.

Ovulation occurs at approximately midcycle, the average time being on the fourteenth day after onset of menstruation. The increased secretion of progesterone that follows the ovulatory process and the formation of the corpus luteum causes a rise in body temperature, which can be used to detect ovulation.

Menstruation as such is not evidence of ovulation. An endometrium grown under estrogen stimulation can bleed either of two methods. If estrogen is withdrawn from a proliferative endometrium, a *withdrawal* type of bleeding usually occurs within 3 days through a process identical with that described previously. Second, if estrogen is administered continuously, bleeding occasionally intervenes on a *breakthrough* basis. These two cases involve an anovulatory cycle.

Many methods of detecting ovulation could be utilized:

1. The increase in body temperature upon progesterone secretion, as mentioned.

2. The change in vaginal cell type has also been widely used as a diagnostic tool.
3. Since both FSH and LH are being secreted at ovulation, the point of maximum hormone titer is also an indication of ovulation.
4. The estimation of products of progesterone metabolism in the urine may be used as a sign of corpus luteum formation, and hence of ovulation.

Still other methods have been proposed.

The extremely delicate balance of the mechanisms of control of FSH, LH, estrogen, and progesterone secretion, together with nervous factors, is well illustrated by the experiments of Everett and Sawyer. They found that ovulation could be blocked in rats by administration of adrenergic blocking agents, but only if the agent was given in a 2-hour time span on the day before ovulation would normally occur. This is only one example of control by the central nervous system, probably the hypothalamus in particular, on the release of gonadotrophin. A direct central nervous system response has long been known in the rabbit, in which the mechanismal stimulation of coitus induces ovulation some hours later. It is also known that suckling of the young, whether or not milk is produced effectively, may inhibit gonadotrophin secretion (presumably FSH). For further discussion of this, see Chapter 4.

The sequence has not been satisfactorily determined experimentally. The exact feedbacks are not known. It is true that, in the postmenopausal woman, the FSH is high and is decreased by estrogen. It is also true that LH levels are decreased by progesterone. However, LH is also decreased by estrogen. The activity of LTH is not well documented; in fact, some investigators believe that LTH may not function in the normal cycle of the human female and may be solely a hormone of pregnancy.

The exquisite sensitivity of this cyclic apparatus shows clearly in the use of birth-control pills. "The pill," which may be estrogens, progestin, or both, alters the proper hormonal concentrations and thus prevents ovulation. It is obvious from the earlier discussion that any interference with the many processes of the cycle could serve as contraceptive measures. These might involve interference with implantation in the prepared uterus (intrauterine device, known as the IUD), dissolution of the ovum or motility of the system (prostaglandins), prevention of ovulation (birth-control pill), and so forth. In fact, all such methods have been tried at one time or another.

ESTROGENS AS SEX HORMONES

The primary endocrine function of the ovary is to maintain the reproductive activity of the organism and to cause the development of the secondary sex characteristics constituting part of the reproductive process. The ovary is inactive in the young girl and begins to produce characteristic secretions only at puberty. The exact mechanism of this awakening is unknown, although some evidence suggests that the immature animal requires only about one-third as much estrogen as the mature animal to produce a given response in the accessory sex organs. Clomiphene will release gonadotrophins from the pituitary *after* puberty, but not before, which suggests that some change in sensitivity of other mechanism occurs at this time. At menarche, the output of gonadotrophin increases. The pituitary secretion at this time is largely FSH, this stimulates the growing follicle to produce estrogen, which is responsible for a large part of the changes in puberty.

The accessory sex organs begin to develop at this time. The fallopian tubes develop in musculature and growth of epithelium, and reach a phase of rhythmic contractions. The uterus develops in musculature by hypertrophy of the muscle cells, and the estrogens increase its contractility. The endometrium of the uterus grows under the influence of estrogen, and the formation of straight tubular glands is stimulated. New enzymes—alkaline phosphatase, for example—appear in the endometrium. There is pronounced growth of blood vessels. The cervical epithelium thickens, and secretory activity begins. There is an increased secretion of mucus from the cervical glands with a decreased fluid viscosity. The vagina develops a tall columnar epithelium with thick walls and cornified cells, and there is a marked deposition of glycogen. The external genitalia develop to adult proportions.

Estrogens also produce the development of secondary sex characteristics. These include the body configuration, deposition of fat, growth of axillary and pubic hair, a typical female hairline, and the cessation of linear growth. Estrogens cause development of the breasts by proliferation of the duct system, but the alveolar system does not grow under this influence.

EFFECTS OF ESTROGENS ON OTHER HORMONES

Estrogen inhibits the release of GH from the pituitary, since animals treated early with estrogen become dwarfed in size and the effect may be overridden by administration of GH. Advantage of this is taken in administering estrogen to young girls who are growing too rapidly in stature. TSH is also affected by estrogen administration, increasing doses of estrogen resulting in decreased TSH production. There is an interesting relationship between the ovary and the adrenal. Female rat adrenal glands are about 60 percent heavier than those of male rats of corresponding size. The adrenal weight of the female can be decreased by castration or administration of androgen. This action of estrogen on the adrenal is not detectable in hypophysectomized animals, indicating an effect on secretion of ACTH. The mouse adrenal-gland cortex has an inner X-zone, which is very large in the female and which disappears under the influence of androgens or pregnancy. The zone persists in the castrated male, but is not demonstrable in the normal male. The human being has a *fetal cortex*, similar to the X-zone of the mouse, which is present in the embryo but which begins to regress soon after birth. It is not known whether the fetal cortex is the result of high titers of estrogen in the mother.

It also appears that small amounts of estrogen are necessary to effect the release of prolactin from the pituitary. High estrogen titers, on the other hand, appear to depress the release of prolactin. This is apparent in pregnancy when the high titers of estrogen prevent prolactin release and milk formation, but after parturition, when the estrogen titer falls, prolactin is released and milk formation begins. Many vitamins, especially folic acid, appear to be necessary for the response of the tissues of the genital tract to estrogens. It has been claimed that the growth of the breasts is stimulated by *mammogens* produced by the anterior pituitary under estrogen stimulation, but the evidence is not clear-cut.

FAILURE OF OVARIAN SECRETION

The normal period of functioning of the female reproductive system is about 35 years. During this time, there are about 450 cycles with an approximately equal number of mature ova formed. Progressive counts indicate that many more ova disappear from the ovary than ever reach maturity. Sections of old ovaries reveal that the cortex becomes thinner, wrinkled, and has fewer follicles as age progresses. There is then a gradual hypofunctioning of the ovary, a decrease in cyclic phenomena, and finally a quiescent ovary. This regression is not due to pituitary failure, for FSH can be detected in large quantities in the urine of women in this stage. There are still follicles in the ovary that show signs of maturation so that the lack of follicles cannot produce the effect. It is possible that the interstitial cells cease to produce estrogen, and indeed the amount of estrogen excreted falls progressively in these individuals. Finally, complete cessation of menstrual cycles and of ovarian function occurs. This is the *menopause*.

In the menopause, there is a progressive degeneration of organs usually maintained by a normal estrogen level. The vagina, the fallopian tubes, and the uterus regress. There may be some regression of secondary sex characteristics, especially in fat distribution and size of the breast.

PROGESTERONE

The reproductive functions of progesterone were summarized in the old name of the hormone *progestin*, accurately called the hormone of gestation, for it prepared the organs of the female for pregnancy. This steroid diminishes the contraction of the myometrium of the uterus; causes growth of glands, vessels, and epithelium of the uterine endometrium, which has been primed by estrogen; decreases the stimulating effect of the estrogens on the vagina and cervix; and causes development of the alveolar system of the breasts after the ducts have been stimulated by estrogen. Some researchers have suggested that parturition occurs because progesterone concentration in uterine muscle decreases, resulting in an increase in uterine contractility.

Most of the secondary female sex characteristics are produced by the action of the estrogens, whereas progesterone serves as the hormone of pregnancy. As a result, the major effect of hypofunction of the ovary is the lack of estrogen. In the immature female, the secondary sex characteristics have not developed, and the normal cyclic phenomena are absent. In the adult, the menstrual cycle ceases in ovarian hypofunction, but there may be little regression of other sex characteristics. The opposite syndrome of ovarian hyperfunction may occur at any age. In the immature, precocity (premature sexual development) develops. High estrogen levels may prevent normal menstrual cycles in the adult. Hypofunction of the corpus luteum usually results in anovulatory cycles, whereas hyperfunction may produce many of the symptoms of pregnancy.

It has been mentioned that the ovary produces two types of hormones from two different endocrine structures. The follicle produces estrogen, and, after rupture of the follicle, the lutein cells produce the second hormone, progesterone, as well as some estrogen. The chemical determination of the metabolites of progesterone indicates that it appears about the same time as the follicle ruptures. In addition to the production of progesterone by the ovary, the placenta secretes large amounts of the steroid during pregnancy. It is well known that the adrenal cortex also produces large amounts of progesterone as precursors of the adrenal corticoids. The testes may also produce this steroid. This is not so well documented, although degradation products of progesterone have been isolated from the testes.

The actions of progesterone outside the reproductive system are few. Progesterone has been reported to cause an increase in body temperature, but it is not at all certain that this is the basis of the 0.3 to 0.5° C rise in basal temperature known to occur at about ovulation. Progesterone effects on metabolism are not clear, except for a pronounced retention of salt and water easily demonstrated in adrenalectomized animals. In large doses, progesterone is androgenic, as would be anticipated from its structure, and will prevent the castration changes in the secondary sex organs of the male. Progesterone probably inhibits LH output by the pituitary; in rats, this is sufficient to prevent ovulation. This antiovulatory action at one time was considered the basis of the array of synthetics with high progesterone activity being used to control human fertility in overpopulated areas.

PREGNANCY

The preparation of the uterus and the ovary for the maintenance of pregnancy has been described. In most cyclic periods, the preparation is wasted. Menstruation reduces the endometrium to basal levels, and the uterus again prepares for the succeeding ovulation. In the human female, fertilization of an ovum released at ovulation, by only one of the many million spermatozoa deposited in the vagina by the male, usually occurs in the fallopian tubes. The fertilized egg then requires about 3 days to descend into the uterus. During this period, the uterus, under the influence of progesterone, is undergoing development into the secretory phase to provide a suitable implantation site. The growing mass of cells from the fertilized egg, the *trophoblast*, may secrete proteolytic enzymes to erode the endometrium to initiate implantation. Implantation cannot be considered to be complete until the erosion or growth has come close enough to a blood vessel so that secretions from the developing placenta can be poured into the mother's bloodstream to maintain the corpus luteum.

The placenta is a remarkable organ designed to maintain the fetus throughout pregnancy. It provides a large exchange surface between the mother and the fetus to permit exchange of gases, food, and waste products. In addition to its role as an exchange organ, the placenta also plays an important endocrine role. (The development of the placenta may be considered a problem of embryology and thus will not be considered here. The same may be said for development of the fetus.)

One of the first signs of pregnancy is the great elevation in gonadotrophin titer circulating in the blood of the mother and excreted in the urine (Figure 12.6). The gonadotrophin, which is produced by the placenta, maintains the corpus luteum and the secretion of progesterone at a time when the pituitary usually ceases to produce LH because of inhibition by the large amounts of circulating progesterone. Human chorionic gonadotrophin is a protein hormone that is largely LH in character, but can exert FSH-like activity in some species of test animals. The titer of gonadotrophin in the blood and

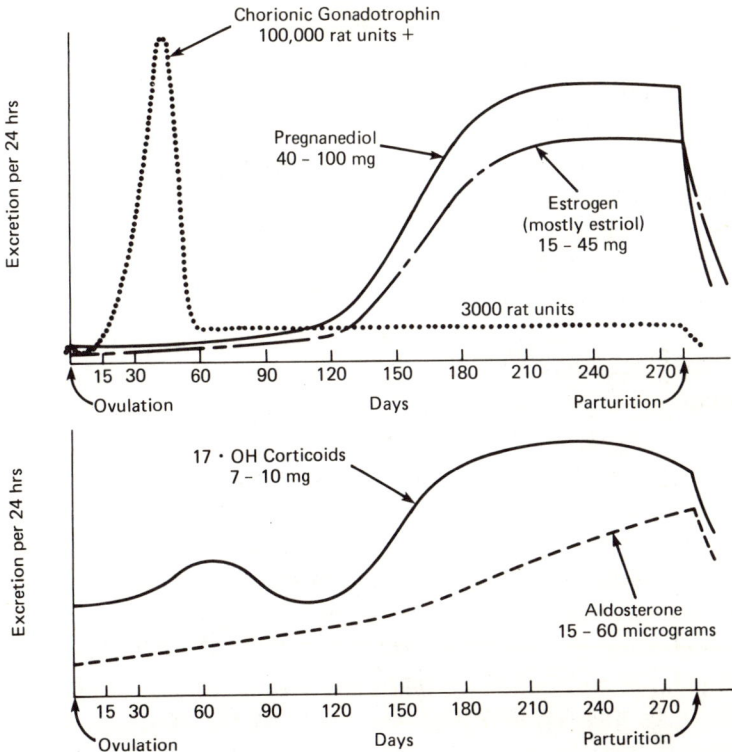

Figure 12.6. The hormonal changes in pregnancy. Note the large placental contribution to the hormone titer.

urine begins to rise almost immediately after fertilization and implantation and reaches a maximum at about 40 days after conception. Tremendous quantities may be produced; titers of 35,000 units per 100 milliliters in the plasma and 250,000 units per day in urinary excretion are not uncommon. The level drops rapidly in 60 to 90 days to about 100 units per day excreted in the urine, and this is maintained throughout pregnancy. Within hours after delivery, the titer drops to almost zero. Maintenance of hormone titer after delivery is the result of failure to deliver all of the placenta, or it may indicate the development of a uterine tumor that secretes the material (chorioepithelioma).

The placenta has been found to be capable of elaborating other protein hormones. Besides gonadotrophin, extracts from placentas have pronounced adrenal- and thyroid-stimulating effects—ACTH and TSH are produced. Placental preparations with appreciable lactogenic and GH activity have been reported, reminding one of the similar situation in human pituitary preparations.

In addition to the protein hormones, the placenta produces steroid hormones. Extracts of placenta have both estrogenic and progestational activity. The secretion of the estrogens and progesterone rises steadily during gestation and drops immediately upon delivery, again suggesting placental rather than ovarian origin (Figure 12.6). Further implication of the placental secretory function is demonstrated by the fact that removal of the ovaries of pregnant women does not prevent the increased titer of both estrogen and progesterone during pregnancy. The fetus is able to protect against high corticoid titers because it possesses the enzymes to convert cortisol to the less potent cortisone but not vise versa, and to convert both to still less potent *tetrahydro-* derivatives. The estrogens probably arise from the fetal adrenal because, when the umbilical cord of the newborn is clamped, estrogen concentration in placental blood drops markedly.

There also is a rise in the excretion of glucocorticoids in the urine during pregnancy. Evidence is accumulating to indicate that much of these may be of placental origin, although there is no doubt that the stress of pregnancy may result in increased output by the adrenal cortex. It has been observed that patients with Addison's disease are capable of excreting large amounts of glucosteroids during pregnancy, and that the adrenal-deficient patient requires less corticoid maintenance during pregnancy; both observations suggest a placental origin of adrenal-like steroids. This is not surprising when the close structural relationship of adrenal steroids to progesterone is recalled. The products of metabolic degradation of the steroid hormones are present in the urine during gestation. The placenta may not produce the same pattern of estrogen secretion as does the ovary, for estriol may comprise 95 percent of the total excreted estrogen during the latter phases of gestation. Most of the estrogen is bound to protein, and it has been suggested that a sudden drop in bound estrogens may be responsible for the initiation of parturition. Progesterone metabolites appear in large enough amounts to be used as an index of pregnancy. The metabolic by-products of adrenal steroids also appear in the urine along with a marked increase in 17-ketosteroids.

It should be emphasized that during the first month or two of pregnancy, the corpus luteum is maintained, and some of the steroids mentioned previously may be secreted by this organ. Following the rapid drop in gonadotrophin production by the placenta, the corpus luteum may regress. In fact, the ovary may be safely removed at this time without interrupting pregnancy, and the placenta takes over the task of producing the necessary hormones during the rest of gestation.

The increased production of estrogen and progesterone during gestation causes characteristic bodily changes. There is a remarkable growth of the uterus in terms of secretory activity of the endometrium as well as in cell size of the muscular wall. The progesterone, in combination with estrogen, appears to exert a depressant effect on the uterus to maintain quiescence. The breasts grow, and the alveolar and duct systems enlarge. There may be production of an opalescent fluid, called *colostrum,* from the breasts, which is somewhat different in composition from milk. Under the influence of estrogen, the cervix becomes softened and enlarged.

The response of the tissues to increased hormone production during pregnancy has not been worked out. Increased plasma protein markedly alters the binding patterns of many hormones, and thus the biological function may not correlate with chemically determined levels.

One of the more common endocrine problems is the diagnosis of pregnancy. Many tests have been developed, and it is outside the scope of this book to present them in detail. Most of the tests are based upon the secretion of increased amounts of gonadotrophin during the early weeks or pregnancy. The *A-Z (Aschheim-Zondek) pregnancy test* is based upon the increase in uterine and ovarian weight of the immature rat when injected with urine from a woman suspected of being pregnant. The *Friedman test* utilizes the formation of small spots that arise on the ovary after ovulation in the urine-injected rabbit as an end point. The *frog test* utilizes the production of eggs or sperm under gonadotrophin stimulation. The *mouse test* is similar to the A-Z test. All of these tests utilize urinary gonadotrophin elaborated by the placenta for assay. New tests have recently been devised for the diagnosis of pregnancy by the antigen-antibody reaction with human chorionic gonadotrophin (HCG) as the antigen. Such tests are now commercially available and can be completed in much less time than earlier procedures.

PARTURITION AND LACTATION

Growth of the fetus and the maintenance of the placenta continue in the human for 10 lunar months (40 weeks). At the end of that time, the fetus and placenta are expelled by the process of *parturition*.

Theories Regarding Initiation of Parturition. The initiation of parturition is not well understood. Several theories have been advanced, but none is adequate to explain completely the beginning of the process.

Estrogen Theory. During about 10 days before termination of pregnancy, the estrogen, which is normally about 95 percent conjugated, suddenly appears in the urine in the free form, and the blood levels of free estrogen may increase 50-fold in a few days immediately preceding parturition. This affords an attractive speculation that the free estrogen increases the motility of the uterus and promotes birth. There is still no explanation for the sudden failure of estrogen conjugation unless it occurs in the placenta, which is aging and which may finally be unable to maintain its previous metabolic activity. These observations in animals have not been confirmed in the human where, in fact, such changes do not occur.

Oxytocin Theory. The posterior pituitary is said to release oxytocic hormone producing contraction of the uterus, which has been sensitized by the free estrogen mentioned previously. A major discrepancy arises, however, because some animals appear to be able to deliver after removal of the posterior pituitary. Furthermore, there is no evidence of increased secretion of oxytocin, although this may not be required if the uterus is rendered sufficiently sensitive to respond to the normal levels.

Placental Theory. The placenta is assumed to elaborate materials that induce labor as they reach sufficient concentrations. The theory is supported by evidence that the placenta produces some highly active oxytocic principle. It is likely that a combination of factors is responsible.

Fetal Theory. If the adrenal and pituitary of the fetus are removed, labor is delayed, thus indicating that some signal from the fetus may trigger the process. Also, the fetal corticoids rise rapidly at the onset of labor, again suggesting a tie-in.

Liggins has proposed the following theory for parturition, which is

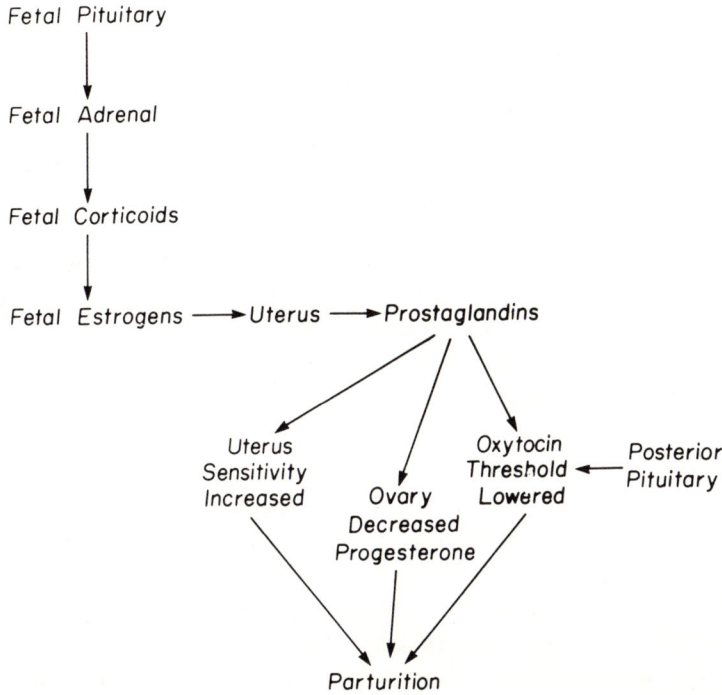

Figure 12.7. The initiation of parturition by the production of fetal hormones.

borne out by measurement of endocrine changes. The fetal adrenal at term begins to produce corticoids. These in turn produce more estrogen by the fetus, because estrogens are an end product of the synthetic cycle. The estrogen stimulates prostaglandin secretion from the uterus, which in turn causes increased myometrial activity. The prostaglandins may also inhibit progesterone production by the placenta, which makes the uterus more sensitive. This initiates contraction (Figure 12.7).

Relaxin. In 1926, Hisaw found that extracts of ovarian tissues, *relaxin*, would cause a relaxation of the *symphysis pubis* of the guinea pig in order to facilitate labor. The hormone is found in greatest quantities in the ovary during pregnancy, although it is also present in the placenta, blood, and urine of the pregnant female. Relaxin is a protein of small molecular weight, and has been obtained in relatively pure form. The concentration rises during pregnancy and disappears immediately after delivery. Recent evidence suggests that the substance may be useful in prevention of premature abortion or labor, as it appears to depress the uterus and retard contractions. Relaxin activity is assayed in arbitrary guinea pig units, consisting of measurement of the degree of widening of the symphysis pubis of the guinea pig followed injection of the desired material. It may also perform the function of widening the birth canal in the pregnant woman as pregnancy advances. Relaxin is probably formed in the ovary and the placenta. The ubiquitous prostaglandins also enter the picture. The prostaglandins can be used to stimulate uterine contraction and have been implicated in the termination of natural pregnancy through antagonism of relaxin.

Lactation. During pregnancy, there is a marked development of the breasts, including growth of the nipple, proliferation of the duct and alveolar system, and production of colostrum. These processes are conditioned by the presence of progesterone and estrogen. Despite the elaborate preparations, the gland does not secrete milk without stimulation from a pituitary hormone, prolactin. The release of prolactin and the production of milk may depend upon the withdrawal of estrogens at parturition, for lactation may be inhibited with large doses of estrogen.

Lactation is induced by the anterior pituitary secretion of prolactin; however, it should not be assumed that this is the only hormone involved in the process, or, for that matter, the only form of stimulation involved (Figure 12.8). Milk synthesis requires the presence of STH and thyroxine (and TSH, indirectly), gluconeogenesis, and protein and fat metabolism, all of which are intimately concerned with mammary gland function. Milk composition and volume also depend upon an adequate supply of vitamins, proteins, carbohydrates, minerals, and the other materials actually entering into the composition of the milk. Milk secretion involves LTH and oxytocin as ejection factors. The flow of milk, once started, is maintained, in part by nervous stimulation from the nipples (see Figure 12.8). Denervation of the nipples prevents formation of milk, but denervation of only one nipple will allow continued milk production in both if the innervated one is suckled. This strongly suggests a hormonal influence, which may be the production of prolactin from the

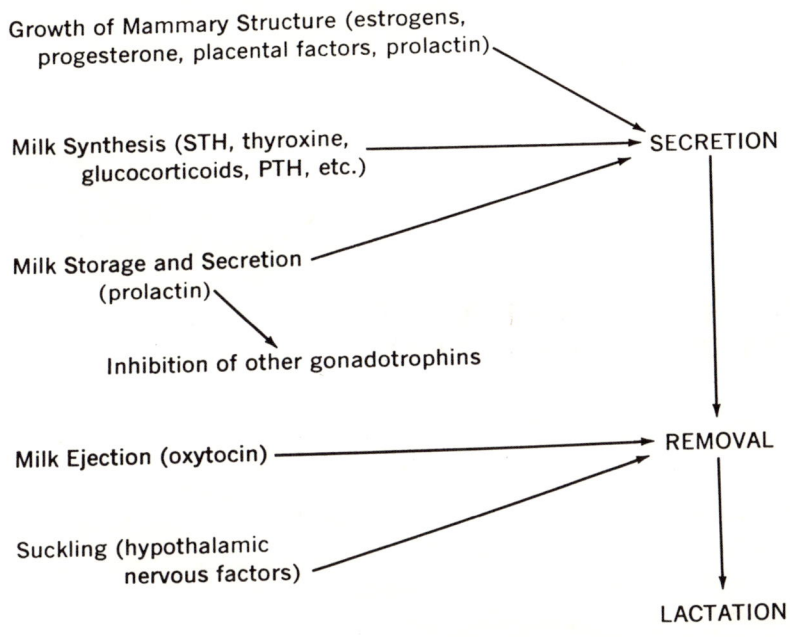

Figure 12.8. The factors influencing lactation.

anterior pituitary stimulated by hypothalamic or other nervous pathways. The function of oxytocin has been discussed previously.

During the period of sucking, the normal menstrual cyclic processes do not usually occur. It is probable that the production of prolactin inhibits the formation or release of other pituitary gonadotrophins and prevents the reestablishment of normal cycles. Inconsistencies in such a process are demonstrated by an occasional pregnancy during active lactation and nursing.

References

Greep, R. O. "Female Reproductive System." *Handbook of Physiology*. Vol. II, Bethesda, Maryland: Amer. Physiol. Soc. 1973.

———. *Reproductive Physiology*. Baltimore: University Park Press, 1974.

Liggins, G. G. *Endocrine Factors in Labor*. London: Cambridge University Press, 1973.

APPENDIX
Control Systems

I. INTRODUCTION

A. *The key principle.* Physiological control systems constantly compare the actual state of the system (i.e , blood pressure) with some reference signal. If an error or diffcience is found, the corrective action is taken automatically.

B. In general, there are two types of feedback systems:
   1) *Regulation feedback.* The reference signal has a constant value. Example: blood sugar regulations.
   2) *Servomechanism feedback.* The reference signal varies. The function of a servomechanism is to insure that the controlled quantity follows, or tracks, the reference signal accurately. Example: proprioceptive muscle servomechanism.
   3) Each of these feedback systems can be one of two types, depending on the sign of the feedback signal at the comparator:
      a) *Negative feedback signal.* Termed *negative* or *degenerative* feedback. Tends to stabilize the controlled quantity and decrease the error signal.
      b) *Positive feedback signal.* Termed *positive* or *regenerative* feedback. Tends to unstabilize the controlled quantity by increasing the size of the error signal. Such systems tend to show oscillations.

II. OPERATION OF A FEEDBACK SYSTEM

A. An increase in the value of the output due to a disturbance acting on the controlled system results in an increase in the signal to the comparator resulting in decreased activity of the effector. When reference signal = feedback signal, the error signal is zero and the effector is inactive.
B. Advantages of feedback:
   1) Control is automatic and requires no conscious effort.
   2) The system resists effects of external disturbances on the controlled system and disturbances in effector function.
   3) Feeding the error signal directly to an effector (gland or muscle, in biological systems; a motor in physical systems) achieves automatic control. This is a feedback system.
C. A given feedback system can serve either as a regulator or servomechanism. The biological elements corresponding to the elements of a feedback system are:

Feedback Element	*Physiological Element*
Reference signals	Nerve impulses, body sensors
Comparator	Hypothalamus
Effector	Releasing factor
Controlled system	Gland
Output quantity	Hormone
Feedback element (sensor)	Changes in body chemistry

D. With the output fixed, the feedback loop can be considered to be functioning as a regulator. An external disturbance tending to displace the output from its fixed position would initiate a sequence of events.

III. FEEDBACK LAG AND OVERSHOOT

A. Due to the delay in signaling the instant the output returned to the rest position, the output may overshoot the rest point, resulting in damped oscillations. In any feedback system, the tendency to exhibit damped oscillations depends on 1) the feedback lag and 2) the rate of response of the effector system.
B. If the rate of response and feedback lag are matched, the system does not overshoot, and we say the system is "critically damped." Most physiological systems show critical damping under usual conditions of operation, with little or no overshoot.

IV. CHARACTERIZATION OF A FEEDBACK SYSTEM: AN ANALYTIC APPROACH TO ILLUSTRATE SOME INTRINSIC PROPERTIES

A. *Component characterization.* Accomplished by use of a transfer function (G), which is defined as a ratio:

$$G_S = \frac{\text{Output}}{\text{Input}} = \text{Transfer function,} \qquad (1)$$

or, for the servomechanism described earlier, we might have:

$$G_S = \frac{\text{Thyroid secretion rate}}{\text{Frequency of action potential in temperature-regulating mechanisms}}. \qquad (2)$$

A simpler system for analysis requiring only algebra might be an electronic amplifier. The transfer function of an amplifier is called its *gain*. It is defined by:

$$\text{Gain } (G) = \frac{\text{Output voltage}}{\text{Input voltage}} = \frac{e_{\text{out}}}{e_{\text{in}}}. \qquad (3)$$

Block diagram notation of an ideal amplifier:

$$e_{\text{in}} \longrightarrow \boxed{G} \xrightarrow{G(e_{\text{in}})} e_{\text{out}}$$

or where $e_{\text{out}} = G(e_{\text{in}})$ by equation (1). \qquad (4)

B. *Open loop systems.*
Block diagram of a nonideal amplifier that is subject to disturbances that affect the output; the output includes the full value of the disturbance, which may either add to or subtract from the gain.

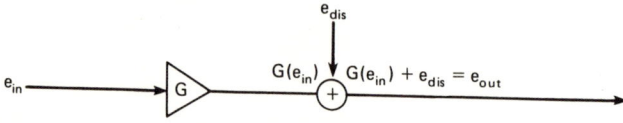

The same system with a fraction F of the output fed back to the amplifier (closed loop).

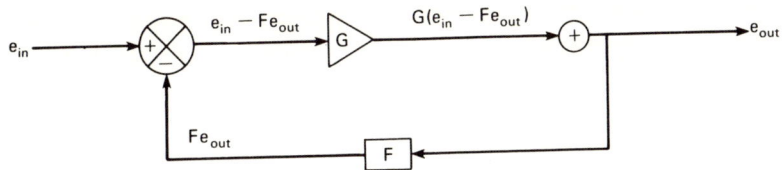

The overall closed-loop gain of this system is still

$$G_{loop} = \frac{e_{out}}{e_{in}},$$

from equation (3). The amplifier gain is:

$$G = \frac{\text{Output}}{\text{Input}} = \frac{\text{Amplifier output}}{\text{Error signal}} = \frac{e_{out} + e_{dis}}{e_{in} + Fe_{out}} \qquad (5)$$

where G = gain, e_{out} = output voltage, e_{dis} = disturbing voltage, e_{in} = input voltage, and F = feedback.

Then: $e_{out} = Ge_{in} - GFe_{out} + e_{dis}$

or: $e_{out}(1 + GF) = Ge_{in} + e_{dis}$

or: $e_{out} = e_{in} \dfrac{(G)}{(1+GF)} + e_{dis} \dfrac{(1)}{(1+GF)}.$ \qquad (6)

In useful feedback systems, the value of G is generally made large and can be on the order of 1 million. The value of F is made close to 1.

C. *Importance of the high gain.*
The participation of e_{dis} in the output is only a fraction.

$\dfrac{(1)}{(1+GF)}$ of its full value. This is particularly true when the outside disturbances do not greatly perturb the system.

When GF is large compared to one, the fraction $\dfrac{G}{1+GF}$ is essentially

$\dfrac{G}{GF}$ or $\dfrac{1}{F}$. Thus, the output is relatively insensitive to changes of G in the amplifier. In physiological systems, effects of effector fatigue are thus minimized.

References

1. Weiner, N. *Cybernetics or Control and Communication in the Animal and the Machine.* 2nd ed. Cambridge: M.I.T. Press, 1962.

2. Houk, J. and E. Henneman. "Feedback control of movement and posture." In V. B. Mountcastle, (ed.), *Medical Physiology*. 12th ed., vol. II. Baltimore: Williams & Wilkins, 1968.
3. Milhorn, M. T., Jr. *The Application of Control Theory to Physiological Systems*. Philadelphia: W. B. Saunders Co. 1965.

Index

Index

Acetylcholine, 62, 135
Acidophilic cells, 43-45
ACTH (adrenocorticotrophic hormone; corticotrophin), 6, 56-58; and adrenal cortex, 5-6, 112-15; and adrenal steroids, 119; and adrenoglomerulotrophin, 128; and aldosterone, 118; assay, 57-58; and biological rhythms, 22; and epinephrine, 130-31; and estrogen, 211; feedback, 121; function, 6, 57-58; and gluconeogenesis, 172; and hypothalamus, 64, 67; and NEFA, 58; and pituitary, 57, 64; and placenta, 215-16; secretion, 121, 130-31; specificity, 2; structure, 56-57; and thyroid, 107
Addison's disease, 57, 216
Adenohypophysis, 43
ADH (antidiuretic hormone; vasopressin), 6, 62, 74-78; action, 75-77; and adrenal steroid deficiency, 127; assay, 78; cellular activity, 31; and cortisol, 113, 115-16; functions, 6, 70, 71, 74-75; and oscillations, 25-26
Adipokinesis, 48-49
Adrenal cortex, 110-11, 111-24; and ACTH, 5-6, 112-15; and adrenal steroids, 112, 113; anatomy, 111-12; and androgens, 119; control, 112-16; and estrogen, 131; hormones, 7; stress, 132-33; structural-functional relationship, 118; and water metabolism, 126-27

Adrenalectomy, 112, 124, 125; effects, 127, 128-31
Adrenal gland, 110-33; anatomy, 110; feedback, 112-13, 118, 140; functions, 110; hormones, 110-11; and testes, 194-195; and thyroid, 131
Adrenalin, 7
Adrenal medulla, 7, 110-11, 134-41, hormones, 134-41; hyperfunction, hypofunction, 140
Adrenal steroids, 116-19; and adrenal cortex, 112, 113; and androgen, 131; assay, 129; and blood sugar, 160; and bone formation, 155; deficiency, 127; form, 12; and hyperglycemia, 171; metabolic paths, 119-28; and stress, 132-33; substitutions, 116-17; synthesis, 119, 120; and thyroid, 107. *See also* Steroids.
Adrenocortical insufficiency, 127
Adrenocortical steroids. *See* Adrenal steroids.
Adrenocorticotrophic hormone. *See* ACTH.
Adrenogenital syndrome, 131
Adrenoglomerulotrophin, 128
Albumin, 119
Aldosterone, 117; and ACTH, 118; action, 128; control, 114-116; effects, 7; and salt metabolism, 126-127
Alloxan, 175
Amino acids, 56-57
Androgen, 187-95; and adrenal cortex, 119;

Androgen (*Continued*)
and adrenal steroids, 131; assay, 189; control, 191-94; extrasexual activity, 195; in female, 190; and FSH, 190; and hypothalamus, 191-93; and ICSH, 60; and insulin, 170; names, 121; production, 187; and prostate gland, 3; and sex, 190-94; as steroids, 116, 187; synthesis, 187-88
Androstendione, 193
Androsterone, 187, 189
Anemia, 129
Angiotensin, 115
Anterior pituitarylike hormone. *See* APL.
Antidiuretic hormone. *See* ADH.
Antihormones, 13
Antiinsulin effect, 124
Antithyroid drugs, 105-06
APL (anterior pituitarylike hormone), 59, 61
Arthritis, 130
Aschheim-Zondek (A-Z) pregnancy test, 217
Assay, 9-11; ACTH, 57-58; ADH, 78; adrenal steroids, 129; androgen, 189; bioassay, 9; catecholamines, 140-41; chemical assay, 9; chorionic gonadotrophins, 61-62; corticoids, 131-32; degradation, 9-11; diabetogenic, 132; eosinophil, 132; epinephrine, 140-41; estrogen, 201-02; FSH, 59-60; GH, 54; glycogen, 131-32, gonadotrophins, 62; hyperthyroidism, 107-09; insulin, 160; LH, 60; MSH, 79-80; ovarian hormones, 201-202; pregnancy, 61-62; progesterone, 201-02; receptor, 35-36; steroid, 122-24, 129; T_4, 109; thyroid, 107-09; TSH, 55-56, 109. *See also* the types of tests.
Asthenia, 129

Barr chromatin pattern, 193
Basal metabolic rate. *See* BMR.
Basophilic cells, 43-45
Bioassay, 9-10. *See also* Assay.
Biological rhythms, 20-26
Blood serum iodide, 91
Blood sugar, 158-60, 162; and energy control, 179-81, 183; level, 4
BMR (basal metabolic rate), 55, 107, 182
Bode plot, 21-22

Bone, 142-56; and adrenalectomy, 130; and estrogen, 2; and hyperthyroidism, 155; and insulin, 145; and parathyroid, 4; metabolism, 143-44
Brain hormones, 7

Calcium, 142-56; control, 144-47; and estrogens, 202; functions, 153-54; ion level, 150; and phosphates, 150-54
Calorigenic activity. *See* Metabolism.
C-AMP (cyclic AMP): and FFA, 184; as mediator, 31-32; and pineal, 82; and prostaglandin, 83, 85; and PTH, 144, 145; and TSH, 93
Carbohydrate metabolism, 158-60, 165-67, 171-73, 202
Carotid, 62, 64
Castration, 190, 194
Catalysts, 2, 4
Catecholamine, 140-41
Cellular activity, of hormones, 29-41
CH (chromatophore hormone). *See* MSH.
Chief cell, 142
Chorionic gonadotrophin, 6, 61-62, 214-15
Chromatography, 9. *See also* Assay.
Chromatophore hormone. *See* MSH.
Chromosomes, 193-94, 198
CIF (corticotrophic inhibiting factor), 112
Circadian rhythm, 82, 206
Circulating thyroid hormone, 95-97, 98-101
Colloid goiter, 105
Contraception, 209-10
Control system, 222-26; amplification, 15; analyses, 17-19; and biological rhythms, 20-26; oscillation, 19-20; theory, 2, 14-15; transfer functions, 16-19
Corpus luteum, 199, 216-17
Corticoids, 24-25; 131-32. *See also* Adrenal gland, hormones; Adrenal steroids.
Corticocosteroids. *See* Adrenal steroids.
Corticosterone, 116-17, 121
Corticotrophic inhibiting factor. *See* CIF.
Corticotrophin-releasing factor. *See* CRF.
Corticotrophin. *See* ACTH.
Cortisol: and ADH, 113, 115-16; binding, 113-19; effects, 7; feedback, 118; and protein, 113; and thyroid, 25
Cortisone, 129, 130

INDEX

Creatine-tolerance test, 109
CRF (corticotrophin-releasing factor), 67, 112-13
Cyclic AMP. *See* C-AMP.
Cytochromes, 93

Damping ratio, 20
Desoxycorticosterone. *See* DOC.
DHT (dihydrotestosterone), 192, 193
Diabetes insipidus, 77-78, 127
Diabetes mellitus, 157-58, 162-67, 177-79; and alloxan, 175; and estrogen, 202; and glucagon, 177; and insulin function, 162; treatment, 174-75
Diabetogenic assay, 132
Dihydrotestosterone. *See* DHT.
DNA, 30, 128
DOC (desoxycorticosterone), 7, 127, 128
Dose-response, 4, 9-10

Electrocorticoids, 129
Enabling action, 6
Endocrine functions, 3, 6-8
Endocrine glands and functions, table, 6-7
Endocrine organs, 3, 12. *See also* the specific organ.
Endocrinologist, 1
Endocrinology, definition, 1
Energy sources, 179-84
Eosinophil, 132
Epinephrine: and ACTH, 130-31, 137; activity, 136-40; assay, 140-41; composition, 6; and glucagon, 176; and glucose, 159-160; and glycogen, 137-39; and homeokinesis, 139; and hyperglycemia, 171; and LH, 137, and muscle fatigue, 138-39; production, 8, 111, 134; tracing, 9; release, 135-36; synthesis, 134-35
EPS (exophthalamus-producing substance), 56
Estradiol, 7, 199, 200
Estriol, 199, 200
Estrogen, 199-206; action, 4, 211; and adrenal cortex, 131; assay, 201-02; and bones, 2; and carbohydrates, 202; cellular activity, 31; and diabetes mellitus, 202; feedback, 202; fetal, 219; and lactation, 220; male, 189, 193; and menstrual cycle, 24, 206-07, 208; and other hormones, 59, 60, 202, 211; and parturition, 218; and pregnancy, 208, 216; and puberty, 210-11; and sex, 2, 210-11; as steroid, 116; types, 199
Estrogen theory, 218
Estrone, 199, 200
Exercise, 179, 183
Exophthalamus-producing substance. *See* EPS.
Exophthalmos, 56

Fast system, 2
Fat metabolism, 171-74, 195, 202, 220
Fatty acids. *See* FFA.
Feedback, 14-15, 26-27, 222-25; and ACTH, 121; and adrenal gland, 112-13, 118, 140; and female endocrinology, 202, 205, 208; and GH, 52-53; and pancreas, 168-69; and starvation, 182-83; and testosterone, 192-93
Female endocrinology, 197-221. *See also* under specific topics.
Female sex hormones, 199-206
Fetal cortex, 112, 194, 211
Fetal theory, 218-19
FFA (fatty acids), 173-74, 181-84. *See also* NEFA.
First messenger system, 31
Follicle-stimulating hormone. *See* FSH.
Free hormone, 118-19
Friedman test, 217
Frog test, 217
FSH (follicle-stimulating hormone), 6, 58-60; and androgen receptors, 190; assay, 59-60; and biological rhythms, 24; and epinephrine, 137; and estrogen, 202; and female cycle, 206-12; and sperm production, 192-94; suppression, 131

Gamma globulins, 129
GAS. *See* General adaptation syndrome.
General adaptation syndrome (GAS), 132-33
Genetic composition, 5
Genotypic abnormalities, 198
GH (growth hormone; STH), 6, 46-50; assay, 54; and biological rhythms, 22-23; and bone, 145, 155; control, 50-55; and estrogen, 211; and glucose, 160, 172-73; and GRF, 51-52; and insulin, 53-54, 170-71; and NEFA, 54; and pituitary,

GH (Continued)
  55-56; and placenta, 216; and somatomedin, 53; and somatostatin, 53, 177
Globulin. See TBG.
Glucagon, 7, 157, 160, 175-81
Glucocorticoids, 129, 216
Gluconeogenesis, 172, 220
Glucose, 158-67, 179-83; blood glucose, 37, 38, 159-60; fat metabolism, 173; and GH, 160, 172-73
Glucose-tolerance curve, 162
Glycogen, 131-132, 137-39
Glycosuria, 162
Goiter, 104-05
Goitrogen, 106
Gonadotrophins, 58-62; assay, 62; and biological rhythms, 24; in males, 3, 191; nervous control, 65; and pituitary, 58-62, 221; and placenta, 217; specificity, 2; types, 58-60. See also Chorionic gonadotrophin; FSH; LH; LTH.
Granulosa, 197
GRF (growth-hormone releasing factor), 51-52

Hair, 130
Halogens, 93
HCF (hyperglycemic glycogenetic factor), 175
HCG (human chorionic gonadotrophin), 59, 61
Holocrine secretion, 8
Homeokinesis, 2, 11-12, 14-15; and adrenal cortex, 130-31; and epinephrine, 139; and insulin, 140; and stress, 132-33
Homeostasis. See Homeokinesis.
Hormonal agents, 70-85
Hormones, 1-13; action, 2-4, 30-33; and cellular activity, 29-41; interrelationships, 36-41; secretion table, 6-7; site of action, 30-33. See also the specific hormones.
Human chorionic gonadotrophin. See HCG.
Hydroquinone, 105
Hyperglycemia, 124, 162, 171, 174
Hyperglycemic agents, 175-77
Hyperglycemic glycogenetic factor. See HCF.
Hyperthyroidism, 56, 95, 107-09, 155
Hypoglycemia, 171, 174, 175

Hypoglycemic agents, oral, 174-175
Hypophysectomy, 112, 124, 190-91, 194
Hypothalamus, 4, 6, 62-68; and ACTH, 64, 67; and androgens, 191-92, 193; and CIF, 112; and CRF, 67, 112; hormones, 31, 62-64; and PG, 84; and pituitary, 42, 43, 62-64, 65; and puberty, 191
Hypothyroidism, 106-09

ICSH (interstitial cell-stimulating hormone). See LH.
Immunochemical assay, 10-11. See also Assay; the specific hormone.
Indoles, 80
Infertility, 190-91
Infrared analysis, 9
Infundibulum, 43
Insulin, 2, 4, 157, 160-74; antibodies, 13; assay, 160; and blood sugar, 160; and bone, 145; and carbohydrates, 165-67; cellular activity, 31; and diabetes mellitus, 162, 177-79; effects, 7, 161-65, 170-74; feedback, 168; form, 12; and GH, 53-54, 170-71; and glucagon, 176-77; and glucose, 165-67; and homeokinesis, 140; and somatostatin, 177; structure, 6, 160
Insulin resistant, 124
Intermediate-lobe hormone. See MSH.
Intermediate lobe, pituitary, 78-80
Intermedin. See MSH.
Interstitial cell-stimulating hormone. See LH.
Iodide, 88-91, 93, 97
Iodide space, 91-92
Iodine, 88-93; activated, 105; deficiency, 93, 95; retention, 94
Islets of Langerhans, 7, 157

Ketosteroids, 131, 189, 190, 193
Kidney, 90, 145, 150-52, 195
Klinefelter's syndrome, 193-94, 198

Lactation, 40, 73-74, 220-21
LATS (long-acting thyroid stimulator), 95
LH (ICSH; luteinizing hormone), 6, 58-60; and androgens, 193; and biological rhythms, 23-24; and epinephrine, 137; and female cycles, 206-07, 209, 214; and hypothalamus, 65; and pituitary, 64; and

INDEX

progesterone, 60, 202, 213; and sex characteristics, 194
Lipogenesis, 125-26
Liver, 7, 159-60, 195, 201
Long-acting thyroid stimulator. *See* LATS.
LTH (luteotrophic hormone; prolactin), 6, 58, 59, 60-61; and biological rhythms, 23, 24; and corticoids, 24-25; and estrogen, 211; and hypothalamus, 65; and lactation, 220-21; and menstrual cycle, 207; and pregnancy, 207-09; and progesterone, 61, 202
Luteinizing hormone. *See* LH.
Luteolytic initiating factor, 84
Luteotrophic hormone. *See* LTH.
Luteotrophin. *See* LH.
Lymphatic system, 129

Maintenance of life assay, 132
Male climacteric, 191
Male endocrinology, 186-96
Mammogens, 211
Masculinization, 119, 121, 132
Mass spectroscopy, 9, *See also* Assay; the specific hormone.
Melanocyte-stimulating hormone. *See* MSH.
Menopause, 191, 194, 212
Menstrual cycle, 203-06, 206-10
Merocrine secretion, 8
Metabolic controls, general, 181-83
Metabolic disease, 119-21
Metabolic hormone. *See* GH.
Metabolism, 2-3, 36-41, 150-55; carbohydrate, 158-60, 165-67, 171-73, 202; and diabetes mellitus, 162-65; and estrogen, 202; fat, 171-74; and glucose, 158-60; salt, 126-27; steroid, 119-31; thyroid control, 101-07; thyroid hormones, 97-98
Methylmercaptoimidazole, 105
Milk ejection effect, 73-74
Morphogenesis, 3
Mouse test, 217
MSH (intermediate lobe hormone; intermedin; melanocyte-stimulating hormone), 7, 57, 78-80
Muscle fatigue, 129, 138-39
Muscle work test, 129

NEFA (nonesterified fatty acids), 54, 58. *See also* FFA.

Neurohormonal glands, 66
Neurohormones, 62, 66
Neurohumors, 62
Neurohypophysis, 6, 43, 70-85
Neurophysine, 71-72
Neurosecretory substances, 62
Nitrogen, 170-71, 195
Nonesterified fatty acids. *See* NEFA.
Noradrenaline, 7
Norepinephrine, 62, 111, 134-41, 184

Obesity, 183
Oocyte, 197, 198
Orinase, 175
Oscillation, control systems, 19-20, 20-22, 24-25
Osmoreceptors, 75
Osteoblasts, 143
Osteoclasts, 143
Osteocytes, 143
Osteoporosis, 195
Ovarian dysgenesis, 194
Ovarian follicle, 197-99, 206-07
Ovary, 197-99; assay, 201-02; hormones of, 7; and PG, 84. *See also* Estrogen; Progesterone.
Ovulation, 84, 208-09
Ovum, 197, 198
Oxyphil cell, 142
Oxytocin, 6, 62, 70-71, 73-74
Oxytocin theory, 218

Pancreas, 157-85; hormones of, 7, 160. *See also* the specific hormones.
Pancreatic tumor, 171
Parathormone. *See* PTH.
Parathyroidectomy, 150-51, 154
Parathyroid glands, 7, 142-43, 154-55
Parathyroid hormone. *See* PTH.
Parturition, 218-20
PBI (protein-bound iodine), 107-08
Perchlorate, 93, 105
Permissive action, 6
PG (prostaglandins), 7, 82-85, 207, 220; PGE, 83-85; PGF, 83-85, 207
Pheochromocytoma, 140
Phosphodiesterase, 93
Phosphorus, 150-54
Pigmentation, 57, 78, 79
Pineal gland, 80-82

Pituitary gland, 42-62; and ACTH, 57, 64; and adrenal cortex, 112; and androgens, 191-92; anterior pituitary, 45-55, 62-64, 199; and biological rhythms, 23; and carbohydrates, 171-73; and castration, 194; hormones of, 3, 6, 7, 45-62, 70-73; intermediate lobe, 78-80; portal system, 62-64; posterior pituitary, 70-85
Pituitary diabetes, 49, 72-73
Pituitary gonadotrophins, 221
Placenta, 61, 214-17
Placental theory, 218
PMS (pregnant mare serum), 59, 61
Polypeptide hormones, 6, 8, 67
Pregnancy, 83, 119, 207-09, 214-17
Pregnancy tests, 61-62
Pregnant mare serum. *See* PMS.
Primary ova. *See* Oocyte.
Progesterone, 7, 199-206, 212-14; assay, 201-02; feedback, 202; and lactation, 220; and LH, 60, 202, 213; and LTH, 61, 202; and ovulation, 208, and PG, 83, 207; and pregnancy, 207-08, 212-13, 216; in testes, 187, 189
Progestin. *See* Progesterone.
Prohormones, 12-13
Prolactin. *See* LTH.
Prostaglandins. *See* PG.
Prostate gland, 3
Protein, 6, 8-9, 30, 113; and lactation, 220, metabolism, 171-73, 202
Protein-bound iodine. *See* PBI.
Protein hormones, 8-9, 10-11, 13
Proteolytic enzymes, 8
PTH (parathyroid hormone, parathormone), 4, 7, 12, 142-43; action, 144; and calcium, 145, 146; and c-AMP, 144-45; and kidney, 150-52; metabolic effects, 154-55; and vitamin D, 148
Puberty, female, 206, 210; male, 190, 191

Radioactive iodide, 92
Radioactive iodine, 108-09
Radioimmunoassay (RIA), 13, 35-36, 58. *See also* Assay.
Radioisotopes, 9
Rebound phenomenon, 191
Receptors, 3-4, 5, 30-34, 35-36
Relaxin, 219-20
Releasing factors (RF), 7

Renal diabetes, 171
Renin, 115-16
RF. *See* Releasing factors.
RIA. *See* Radioimmunoassay.
Ring structure, 6

Salt metabolism, 126-27
Sayers test, 57
Secondary spermatocytes, 186
Second messenger system, 31
Sella turcica, 43
Serotonin, 7
Sertoli cells, 186-87, 193
Serum cholesterol level, 109
Sex characteristics, 3, 190, 193-94, 210-11
Sex hormones, 2, 195. *See also* the specific hormones.
Skin, 130
Slow system, 2
Sodium, 17-18, 18-19
Somatomedin, 7, 53
Somatostatin, 7, 53, 177
Somatrophic (growth) hormone. *See* STH.
Sperm, 187, 192-94
Spermatids, 186-87
Spermatogenic cells, 186
Sphenoid bone, 43
Spiralactone, 128
Spontaneous defects, 5
Starvation, 179-81, 181-83
Sterility, 190
Steroids, 8-9; assay, 122-24, 129; by corpus luteum, 216-17; metabolism, 119-31; of placenta, 216; structure, 116
Steroid diabetes. *See* Hyperglycemia.
STH (somatotrophic, or growth, hormone), 220
Stress, 3, 130-33, 135-37, 140
Sulfa, 105
Sulfation factor. *See* Somatomedin.
Sulfonylurea, 175
Supraoptic nucleus, 71

Tachyphylaxis, 75
Target organ, 3, 4
TBG (thyroxine-binding globulin), 95-96
TBP (thyroxine-binding protein), 95-96
TBPA (thyroxine-binding prealbumin), 95-96
TCT (thyrocalcitonin), 7, 143, 145-46, 155-56

INDEX 235

Testes, 3, 7, 186-89, 194-95
Testosterone, 2, 7, 131, 187; and androsterone, 189; and estrogen, 189, 193; feedback, 192-93; and ICSH, 192
T_4 (thyroxine), 7, 9, 94, 95; assay, 109; and cellular function, 106; and circulating thyroid hormone, 95-97; control, 98-101; iodine in, 91; and lactation, 220; and metabolism, 97-98, 101-05; and TSH, 106
Theophylline, 83, 93
Thiamylal, 105
Thiobarbiturates, 105
Thiocyanate, 93, 105
Thiopental, 105
Thiouracil, 91, 92, 105
Thiourea, 105
Thyrocalcitonin. See TCT.
Thyroglobulin, 8, 13
Thyroid, 3, 7, 87-109; and ACTH, 107; activity table, 104; and adrenal gland, 131; and adrenal steroids, 107; assay, 107-09; and castration, 194; and cortisol, 25; hormones, 4, 8, 12-13, 88-93, 93-105; and TSH, 2, 55, 92-93, 98. See also Circulating thyroid hormone; T_4; T_3.
Thyroid iodide, 91
Thyroid-stimulating hormone. See TSH.
Thyroid-to-serum-iodine ratio. See T/S.
Thyronine, 94
Thyrotrophin. See TSH.
Thyroxine. See T_4.
Thyroxine-binding globulin. See TBG.
Thyroxine-binding prealbumin. See TBPA.
Thyroxine-binding protein. See TBP.
Transcortin, 119
Transfer functions, control system, 16-19

Triiodothyronine. See T_3.
TRIT. See T_3.
Trophic hormones, 3, 46-55, 62
Trophin hormones. See Trophic hormones.
Tryptophan, 80, 82
T/S (thyroid-to-serum-iodine ratio), 91, 93
TSH (thyroid-stimulating hormone; thyrotrophin), 2, 6, 55, 98-106; and ACTH, 107; assays, 55-56; and c-AMP, 93; and circulating thyroid hormone, 96; and female system, 211, 216, 220; and hyperthyroidism, 95; and pituitary, 55-56; and radioactive iodide, 92; and T_4, 106; and thryoid, 2, 55, 92-93, 98; and T_3, 106
T_3 (triiodothyronine; TRIT), 7, 94-98, 106; assay, 55-56, 109; iodine in, 91
T_3/T_4 ratio, 93
Turner's syndrome, 198
Tyrosine, 93

USP (US Pharmacopeia) unit, 56
US Pharmacopeia. See USP.
Uterus, 73. See also the specific functions.

Vascular system, and stress, 132-33
Vasoconstriction, 139
Vasodilation, 139
Vasopressin. See ADH.
Vitamin D, 144, 145, 147-50

Water metabolism, 126-27
Water retention, 127

Zona fasciculata, 112, 118
Zona glomerulosa, 112
Zona reticularis, 112, 118